THE NATURAL WAY TO A HEALTHY SKIN

THE NATURAL WAY
TO A HEALTHY SKIN
by the Editors of Prevention Magazine

COMPILED by

ROBERT BAHR

EDITED by

CHARLES GERRAS

and

JOAN BINGHAM

RODALE PRESS, INC.

EMMAUS, PENNA. 18049

PUBLISHED BY RODALE PRESS BOOK DIVISION
33 EAST MINOR STREET, EMMAUS, PENNA. 18049

FIRST PRINTING NOVEMBER, 1972
PB-106
SBN 0-87857-047-0

LIBRARY OF CONGRESS CATALOGUE CARD NUMBER:
72-84795
MANUFACTURED IN THE UNITED STATES OF AMERICA

Contents

Chapter

I	The Miracle of Your Skin	1
II	Nutrition and Common Sense	10
III	The (Vitamin) ABC's of Healthy Skin	22
IV	The Skin As A Warning Device	32
V	Are You Photosensitive?	35
VI	The Myth of the Healthy Tan	41
VII	Sweat To Save Your Life	52
VIII	The Mystery Rashes	59
IX	Prickly Heat	79
X	Burns	83
XI	Shingles	94
XII	Acne	103
XIII	Athlete's Foot	113
XIV	Eczema	117
XV	Ichthyosis and Psoriasis	124
XVI	Vitiligo	135
XVII	Warts	139
XVIII	Drugs and Your Skin	143
XIX	Young Skin Forever	150
XX	Cosmetics	156
XXI	Hair	168
XXII	The Natural Beauty Plan	178

[v]

Chapter I

The Miracle of Your Skin

There's probably no organ in the body that is taken more for granted than the skin. Virtually everyone has pondered the tragedy of losing his eyesight, has plugged his fingers in his ears to conceive to some extent what it would be like to be deaf. We've all thought about heart attacks, strokes, and most of us have even wondered at least once about mental illness, a malfunctioning brain.

But unless the skin gives us problems, we tend to ignore it with the unconscious assumption, "Sure I have skin. It's a sac into which my body has been poured. So what?" That attitude is naive, of course. The skin does a great deal more than hold us together. Some of its functions are so important that without them we would surely die.

But the consequences of the ignorance most of us display toward the functions of the skin are very serious. Because we take the skin for granted, we tend to be unaware of its unique needs and the care it requires. Because of this, skin problems have become practically universal. Acne is so widespread among teenagers that they have come to think of it as a normal fact of life. Additional millions have skin reactions due to allergies. Eczema, ichthyosis, psoriasis, and other skin ailments are very widespread. Medical authorities estimate that more than 115,000 Americans will contract skin cancer this year. According to the *American Dermatological Society,* an astounding number of Americans are suffering from contact dermatitis, the skin's adverse reaction to chemicals in clothing and other materials.

Usually these ailments can be prevented; and if they have already occurred, they can be cured. As W. A. Krehl, M.D., Ph.D., points out in *The Medical Clinics of North America* (September, 1964), skin ailments are often a reflection of nutritional deficiency. A dry, scaly skin suggests a vitamin A shortage. Cracked, inflamed tissue around the nose and lips is a strong hint that the intake of the B vitamins pyridoxine and riboflavin are inadequate. Eczema in an infant is often nothing more than a lack of essential fatty acids in his diet. A skin that tends to bruise probably means weak capillaries, a common result of vitamin C and bioflavonoid insufficiency. As Dr. Krehl puts it, "The skin is very frequently an early barometer of inadequate nutritional status."

Many skin blotches, rashes, itches and inflammations result from a contact dermatitis. Others may be caused by foods, or by some drugs. Air pollution is sometimes responsible for serious skin problems.

With sufficient knowledge of the skin, even susceptible individuals can prevent ailments such as these. Unfortunately, most of us neglect the skin until it gives us trouble.

[2]

Actually, the skin we treat so carelessly is the largest organ of the body; it weighs about twice as much as the liver and covers a total area of more than 21 square feet for most of us. We rely on the skin to adapt our systems to changes in temperature and humidity, so that we can survive the below-freezing cold of a winter's day, or the 200-degree heat we are exposed to in a sauna. The skin must function efficiently to maintain our inner temperature at a stable 98.6 degrees F. Any severe fluctuation in this temperature can be fatal.

It is the skin that has the major responsibility for warding off infectious organisms. The skin is continually exuding wastes from our bodies. It puts up with caustic chemicals, such as washing fluids and a wide variety of other irritants. It takes the brunt of bruises, scratches and blows. It is an extremely tough fabric, and at the same time, very resilient and flexible. It is soft and warm to the touch, and when well cared for, satin-smooth.

The body depends on skin to warn of danger. Its incredibly complex network of nerves report promptly to the brain's central control the presence of heat, cold, pressure and pain.

In his book, *New Hope For Your Skin,* Irwin I. Lubowe, M.D., reports that each square inch of skin contains:

78 nerves
650 sweat glands
19 or 20 blood vessels
78 sensory apparatuses for heat
13 sensory apparatuses for cold

[3]

1,300 nerve endings to record pain

19,500 sensory cells at the ends of nerve fibers

160 to 165 pressure apparatuses for the sense of touch

95 to 100 sebaceous glands

65 hairs and muscles

19,500,000,000 cells

There are three layers to the skin—the epidermis or surface layer, the dermis, or true skin, and the sub-dermis, where most of the activity of the skin is carried out.

The top layer of skin, the epidermis, is actually dead skin, for the most part. These skin cells have shriveled up into flat plates. The nuclei have vanished, and all that is left is a horny material. In some ways it's roughly comparable to the scales of a fish—and it has the same function: to protect the layers of skin beneath. This is why the human body can sustain so many bumps and bangs. When a bruise does develop, it means that the underlying layers of skin have been damaged to the point where some bleeding has occurred. Without the epidermis, a minor injury would result in actual bleeding. The horny layer contains the injury and prevents much more serious damage.

Sometimes this outer layer is rubbed away faster than it can be replaced by the constantly maturing cells beneath it. It is natural for these cells to fall away, but if we hasten the process through excessive friction, the result is a blister. The epidermal cells have a way of coping with that problem, if it recurs frequently, by

[4]

forming an extra-thick horny layer over the area that gets too much use—a callous. Sometimes these develop in undesirable areas, such as the bottom of the foot, and can cause a great deal of pain. (In such cases, a doctor can shave the callous quickly and easily—but because the growth may be something other than a callous, it should be removed only by a physician. Too many do-it-yourself surgeons have developed a serious infection, or incurred serious bleeding while attempting a simple operation of this sort.)

The epidermis is also responsible for producing hair follicles, sweat glands, the nails and the sebaceous glands. The sebaceous glands produce sebum, a kind of spontaneous face cream, which contains waxes and fatty acids that destroy or inhibit the growth of germs on the skin. The sebaceous glands are found in every part of the skin except the palms, soles of the feet, fingernails and toenails. They are particularly plentiful around the nose, cheeks, mouth and chin, where they can be particularly useful in trapping viruses and bacteria that would enter the nasal and oral cavities.

Sometimes the sebum does its job of trapping dirt so effectively that it forms a plug across the sebaceous glands. The result is a blackhead, or a whitehead. There are effective ways to cope with this problem, and we will discuss them at length in later chapters. But the fact is that sebum—composed of acids and salts as well as oil, water, and old skin cells—is the miracle of nature, essential for soft, smooth and healthy skin.

Other important functions of the epidermis are to produce fingernails, toenails and hair. Says Reginald

[5]

T. Brain, M.D., in his book *Skin Diseases*, "Hair roots are formed by collections of specialized epidermal cells arranged as a cone, and these cells go through the changes of producing horny material just like the other epidermal cells. The hairs are built up from round flat horny cells like little carved tiles around the central core of less organized material called the medulla of the hair. Pigment is deposited into these cells and this accounts for the blond or brunette, according to the amount of dark pigment the hair contains. As the cylindrical hair shaft is formed it is pushed upwards and runs between sheets of cells partly formed from the hair root and partly from the walls of the hair bulb or follicle which supports the hair in its progress from the root to the skin surface." When the hair is finally made, it is simply a pile of dead horny skin cellls

It is the same with nails. "The epidermis produces a cleft from which modified and closely-packed horny cells emerge as the fingernail plate. The nail plate is just as dead as the hair, but it is derived from actively growing cells richly supplied with blood vessels and nerves and the nail plate is firmly and intimately attached to the nail bed or matrix throughout most of its length."

Beneath the epidermis is the dermis, a jelly-like substance through which runs the nerves, blood vessels, roots of the sweat and sebaceous glands and a few random tissue fibers. This dermal layer is referred to as the "true skin" because here alone is the living skin tissue. It is the dermal layer of the skin which must be protected from the outside environment, and it is also

[6]

this layer which must be supplied adequately with nutrients by the blood stream.

The dermal layer of the skin differs greatly from the epidermal layer: it is far more sensitive than the dead horny cells on the body's surface; well supplied with blood vessels, it will bleed easily from even a slight injury; and if its nutritional needs are not met precisely, it will develop an adverse reaction.

Dr. Daphney A. Roe, M.D., of Cornell University Graduate School of Nutrition, Sage Hospital, says that, the dermal layer of the skin "reflects the well-being or the disorders of the organism. It is a turbulent tissue and it grows, differentiates and renews itself at all times." Because of that sensitivity, "In man, as in other animal species, the skin is a mirror of the nutritional status and evidence of the malnutrition can be obtained from proper observation not only of the skin, but also of associated structures such as hair and nails."

The nutrients we eat are absorbed by the blood stream and reach the skin by means of capillaries, the smallest blood vessels found in the body. Nutrition is just as important for the skin as it is for any other organ of the body. A healthy skin is one of the dividends of a healthful diet.

The proper growth of the dermal cells insures the skin against injury and infection. The preservation of an intact horny layer, the production of an oily surface film, and the secretion of an acidic sweat, are functions completely dependent upon the growth of these cells. An adequate supply of protein is essential for a beauti-

[7]

ful skin, says Dr. Roe, because without it, dryness results, and the skin loses its defense against infection, sunlight, wind, and cold.

When the diet is deficient in some particular nutrient a symptom of that deficiency usually ensues. A skin oversensitive to light is a recognizable sign of a niacin (vitamin B_3) deficiency. Though pellagra, a sometimes fatal disease due to a niacin deficiency, was once quite prevalent, it is rather uncommon today, but marginal deficiencies of niacin still frequently lead to symptoms resembling pellagra. Typical of these is a rash similar to prickly heat which usually appears on the neck, forearms, and other uncovered parts of the body. The skin is dry, somewhat scaly, and shows fine wrinkles and a coarse texture.

Fissures or cracks at the angles of the mouth are the common result of a deficiency in riboflavin (vitamin B_2). These ugly and painful cracks in the skin's surface may become chronic if the deficiency persists for too long. This weakens the skin's ability to protect itself against infections.

The skin, by its very nature, is designed to maintain itself, to stay healthy, fresh, and attractive. Damaged tissues merely disappear as new ones take their place, even into the later years.

When the skin doesn't work this way, the blame can usually be put on an inadequate supply of the nutrients the skin needs to function properly. People who carefully avoid poisons that might destroy their kidneys or liver, and wouldn't dream of deliberately damaging their noses or ears, unknowingly subject their skin to

[8]

chemicals which are ruinous to it. Skin problems are usually the product of ignorance. The first big step to a healthy skin is an appreciation of what skin is all about.

Chapter II

Nutrition and Common Sense

The program of skin care we advocate in this book can be summarized in four simple words—NUTRITION AND COMMON SENSE. There is no better way to improve the skin and keep it looking and functioning well.

"Adequate nutrition is essential for the preservation of a healthy skin just as it is essential for the maintenance of a healthy body. So it is not surprising that the skin is one of the first and major sites in which vitamin deficiencies manifest themselves." This is the opinion of Drs. Rudolph Baer and Sheldon Brodie of New York University, as expressed in *The Practitioner*. The two researchers describe the ways various vitamin deficiencies show up on the skin. "The skin of patients suffering from vitamin A deficiency," for example, "generally tends to be dry, scaly and crinkled, and sometimes has the fishskin-like appearance of ichthyosis."

"Riboflavin (vitamin B$_2$) deficiency presents characteristic cutaneous (skin) mucous membrane changes. Here one may see cheilosis with reddening, thinning, scaling, chapping and wrinkling of the lips . . . "

Vitamin C deficiency, in its early stages, manifests itself in "hyperkeratoic follicular papules on the but-

[10]

tocks and calves," eventually leading to scurvy. (See "The [Vitamin] A,B,C'S of Healthy Skin" for a complete discussion of the role vitamins in skin health.)

Can we defend against such vitamin-deficiency problems by merely ingesting the so-called "minimum daily requirement" of each vitamin to protect us? Not according to Baer and Brodie who insist, "the possibility must be considered that the individual or his skin may require a higher level for vitamins or for a specific vitamin than that which is generally accepted by nutrition experts as 'normal.' In some patients such unusually high requirements for vitamins appear to be due to a metabolic peculiarity or the result of infection, pregnancy, or a systemic disease. Still another condition which may account for avitaminosis, but which thus far has received little attention, is the role of the vitamin competitors (chemicals and other substances which destroy vitamins) . . . There seems, however, to be limited knowledge concerning the natural occurrence of such competitors in food and especially in the form of additives in modern 'prepared' foods and in drugs."

Many teenagers continue to suffer the social embarrassment and frequent permanent scarring of acne, even though sufficient medical evidence exists showing that this youthful skin disorder often responds quickly to vitamin A therapy.

The vitamins of the B complex have also been used with great success in treating skin diseases.

In recent years, significant evidence has accumulated that unsaturated fats and proteins play impor-

[11]

tant roles in maintaining healthy skin. Now we know that deficiencies in either of these nutrients can lead to a host of skin ailments.

The Unsaturated Fatty Acids

Unsaturated fatty acids come from vegetable oils that stay liquid at room temperatures—the kind of oils you use, for example, in salad dressings, or eat in nuts and avocados without even knowing it. What happens if you are placed on a diet free of the unsaturated fatty acids?

Among other things, you might be inviting skin trouble. Drs. Worne and Schneider, writing in the medical journal, *Archives of Research,* describe the state of 24 gall bladder patients who had been on a fat-free diet (less than one percent of their daily calories was in the form of fat) for a year or longer. The two researchers tested the blood of these patients for fatty acid content. It was well below normal. All of the subjects suffered from "a dry, flaky skin, threaded with fine lines and wrinkles." There was also a slight to moderate itching in most cases.

They were given a cream containing unsaturated fatty acids and told to apply it to the affected areas every night and morning. Results were excellent, speedy and apparently without any unpleasant side effects. The product used in this experiment is probably not available commercially, but if you suffer from the conditions mentioned above, you might ask your doc-

[12]

tor to prescribe a cream or salve containing unsaturated fatty acids.

The connection between unsaturated fatty acids and skin health is clearly demonstrated in laboratory experiments. Animals on a fat-free diet develop a condition called fat-deficiency disease. Rats show arrested or retarded growth, changes in skin and hair, kidney disorders, impairment of reproductive function and a raised metabolic rate. This means that they burn up their food more rapidly.

The skin of these animals becomes dry and scaly and covered with dandruff. Cold weather accentuates the condition. Just adding fats—any kinds of fats—to the diet of these animals does not improve the condition. But adding unsaturated fats, chiefly linoleic and linolenic acids, reverses the process and cures the skin conditions.

(It is noteworthy that human breast milk is rich in unsaturated fatty acids—far richer than cow's milk. Could it be that the American aversion to breast feeding has something to do with the prevalence of eczema among our infants and children? Certainly the fact that human breast milk is rich in unsaturated fatty acids indicates that these are essential for the new baby or they would not be provided by nature in such abundance. Where do children who are not breast fed obtain these valuable fats?)

An article in *Munchener Medizinische Wochenschrift (Munich Medical Weekly)*, Vol. 26, p. 1308, 1961, discusses the work of Dr. Sigwald Bommer who used various unsaturated fats in treating eczema and other skin conditions—psoriasis, boils and certain kinds of ulcers. He tells us that these fats in the diet have a direct, if mysterious, effect on the function of blood vessels and circulation. He believes that people today get too much of the saturated fats and too little of the unsaturated ones.

Dr. Bommer reports on 6 years of his own experience in giving oils rich in unsaturated fats to his patients. It is certain, he says, "and has been substantiated by observation, especially in children, that too great a restriction of the total supply of fat reacts definitely also on the skin and can produce pathological changes (impetigo, eczema, etc.). In connection with this, it is interesting to know that Norwegian breeders of furred animals feed linseed cakes to their silver foxes in order that these animals may grow an especially beautiful coat of fur."

Believing that vitamin E would aid in the treatment of his experimental patients, Dr. Bommer added it, but saw no significant improvement. However, when he changed to wheat germ oil (rich in vitamin E), there was an immediate difference. The question arose: was it the vitamin E or the unsaturated fats in the wheat germ that brought about the improvement? Whatever the answer, the wheat germ oil did get results.

Three other researchers have reported good results in treating boils with unsaturated fats, says Dr. Bommer. Linoleic and linolenic acids (both present in the various oils we mentioned above) were used. (Dr. Bommer treats these patients with a diet completely free of sweets, canned fish and meat, including sau-

[14]

sages. The diet is supplemented with vitamin C and vitamin A.)

Blood tests of psoriasis patients show that levels of unsaturated fats are 20 to 50 percent lower than in healthy persons. Dr. Bommer gave wheat germ oil preparation to one patient who was completely cured of psoriasis of several years' duration within a few weeks. Other patients did not find this complete relief. At present, Dr. Bommer gives folic acid (a B vitamin) for psoriasis.

He also uses vegetable oils for treating ulcers externally—leg ulcers specifically. This oil, he says, is far superior to other local preparations for ulcers. He still does not know, he says whether it is the vitamin E or the unsaturated fats which do the work. Using an unsaturated fat preparation, he obtained "surprisingly rapid granulation and regeneration of the skin, even where there were many ulcers and several of a considerable size. The ointment is also well tolerated by a sensitive skin."

Dr. Bommer recommends the unsaturated fats treatment both internally and externally for infantile eczema and the ezcema that older children and adults may have, which comes from some systemic cause, not from an allergy.

There seems to be little doubt that the good health of the skin is closely tied in with the fat content of the diet. One needs to get enough of the unsaturated fats and not too much of the saturated ones.

How do you use these unsaturated oils? You can, of

course, take them in a spoon like medicine, but why do this, since they are foods and very pleasant, agreeable foods too. Why not pour them over your salads mixed with a little vinegar or lemon juice, plus herbs, garlic or whatever else you like for seasoning? Use liquid oils whenever you use fats in cooking. It is wise to shun all fats that are solid at room temperature. These include all margarines and the solid white shortenings used for baking, as well as meat fats and butter. Saturated fats are almost universally used in the processing of foods, so avoid processed foods, such as crackers, precooked TV dinners, rolls and muffin mixes, cake mixes, bakery products and so forth. Prepare your own food in your own kitchen.

Protein vs. Wrinkles

Protein foods might solve the problem of wrinkles, according to a report by Dr. Charles S. Davidson of Harvard Medical School and Boston City Hospital. He told a symposium on various aspects of old age that the glands may play the largest part in this so-called "withering" process. With age the glands gradually decrease their functioning, making less and less protein available for the skin, muscles and other organs. But, older people tend to eat less protein, perhaps this is responsible for the glands slowing down followed by the wrinkling of the skin. If you would avoid wrinkles, keep your diet high in protein and low in carbohydrates to give your glands every opportunity to function healthfully. Your glands and your skin are made

[16]

of protein; a high-protein diet should help to keep them in good repair.

Sunflower seeds seem to have a healthful effect on the skin. We don't know why. It may be because they are high in protein, or because they contain considerable amounts of the B vitamins and vitamin A. Just like peanuts or popcorn, one handful of sunflower seeds leads to another. It's perfectly all right to eat as much as you want of this healthful food, but if you are on a reducing diet, remember that the seeds are rich in calories.

The nutritional program we will advocate in this book is one which can keep the skin in optimum health. Although we will go into it in much greater detail hereafter, here is the nutritional program in a nutshell:

Maintain a well-balanced diet containing fresh fruits, and vegetables (a good percentage of them raw, and organically-grown whenever possible), meat, seeds and nuts.

In addition, be sure to include a full program of food supplementation, including fish oil capsules for vitamin A, brewer's yeast and desiccated liver for the B complex, and rose hips or acerola for vitamin C. Of course, all the other vitamins and minerals are important too; nutrients work best in concert to promote general health.

But nutrition, although it is of great importance, is only half of our program.

Because the skin is man's major contact with his environment, this six pounds (on the average) of com-

[17]

plex tissue receives the brunt of outside abuses. It needs sensible protection from the outside.

Thus, the second part of our program—common sense—calls for avoiding those substances which irritate the skin from the outside. It sounds simpler than it is, at least for some people. These are the ones who get their medical advice from TV commercials. They are convinced that the answer to all skin problems is to kill bacteria with soap. Actually, the excessive use of soap irritates the skin so much that further breaks in the skin results, opening the gates for a whole new batch of bacteria to pour in. Most of us can get really clean by gently rubbing with a wash cloth soaked in plain, warm water.

Too many skin disorders that need professional attention are aggravated by "over-the-fence" medical advice.

Well-meaning neighbors who wouldn't dream of prescribing a drug for you to take, will casually pass on to you half a tube of "that stuff" the doctor ordered for her skin disorder. "It'll cure anything."

Another harsh irritant to the skin is one to which millions wilfully subject themselves every summer. To many of us, the golden-brown suntan is a hallmark of health. We have no idea why. Excessive exposure to the sun (and when exposure is enough to change the skin's color, it is excessive) causes premature aging of the skin, unsightly blotches, a tough, leathery texture, and can even lead to skin cancers. It seems that the world has turned from the ivory-skinned ideal to the bronzed idol.

[18]

The first thing to do when a skin irritation appears is to throw out all your old skin remedies. There must be something which is causing the irritation. Try to track it down. That new wool sweater may be causing the rash on your shoulder, or maybe it's the soap you are using. Itching ears may be traced to new earrings; itching scalp can result from anything used on the hair. Rings can make fingers sore; shoes can react badly with the feet.

If the problem persists after two weeks, see your doctor. Meanwhile an icebag applied to the area will help to relieve itching, so will cornstarch applied as a dusting powder. Of course, swelling, spreading, bleeding, or infections and sharp injuries to the skin, call for immediate medical attention.

So here we have two keys to a healthy skin: nutrition, and common sense. Avoid refined foods and saturated fats, and keep the body well supplied with nutrients through a balanced diet rich in all vitamins, plus a regular intake of food supplements to maintain a good supply.

Treat the skin as an organ, worthy of the best care. Avoid irritants, especially strong soap, harsh cosmetics, and prolonged exposure to the sun. The skin is the mirror of your body's health. Keep it healthy inside and out.

Emotions Affect Your Skin, Too

Skin disorders may proceed from emotional causes, says Dr. D. Cappon, writing in the *Canadian Medical*

[19]

Association Journal. His views are based on some 40 actual case histories from his own files and those of his fellow-doctors. The article presents evidence that skin symptoms—all the way from blushing to psoriasis —are sometimes rooted in the emotions. Dr. Cappon says that holding-in certain emotions may produce hives. He gives as examples: a convict who developed hives daily just at the time he was locked in his cell after the day's exercise period; a manufacturer who developed an itching skin as he watched his factory burn to the ground; a woman who developed hives whenever she became angry with her husband in social situations where she could not scold him.

Persons with asthma-eczema-itch complex are often apt to be "over-anxious, needing to excel, above average in intelligence, overdependent and overprotected" says Dr. Cappon. Sexual maladjustment, hatred of a cruel parent, or a personality withdrawn into imaginary life often produce these conditions, he says. Fever blisters and cold sores sometimes follow emotional upsets in patients who are usually submissive, obedient and sweet. Outbreaks of psoriasis also may be related to emotional disturbances, according to Dr. Cappon.

Why talk about emotions in a chapter about nutrition? More and more psychiatric researchers are coming to believe that emotional states are largely biochemical in origin. Schizophrenia is being treated with niacin (vitamin B_3). Personality disturbances, even insanity, are among the symptoms of pellagra, a dis-

[20]

ease caused by vitamin B deficiency. So a nutritionally adequate diet might do as much or more to treat emotionally induced skin problems than an analyst can.

Chapter III

The (Vitamin) ABC's of Healthy Skin

Vitamin A

For more than thirty years now, the medical community has been studiously neglecting the role vitamins play in maintaining health. In the process, it has been "forgetting" priceless information which was wisely utilized in the past to keep people healthy.

Now there is evidence that this trend is reversing— at least with vitamin A. In December, 1968, a leading nutritional authority tossed a live grenade to those doctors who have been advising reduction in vitamin A intake, when he quietly but assuredly stated that humans cannot effectively resist infections of many kinds unless their vitamin A reserve is high

The authority was Dr. George Wolf, a professor at the Massachusetts Institute of Technology. Last fall he conducted an international symposium on vitamin A at the MIT campus. He is a shy, soft-spoken man, apparently determined to reverse the damage done by misguided medical men who are suspicious of a nutrient essential to life. For the attending doctors, there was dynamite in the simple affirmation that "Vitamin

[22]

A may properly be referred to as the anti-infection vitamin."

Speaking at the 135th annual meeting of the American Association for the Advancement of Science, Dr. Wolf also named three other necessary functions vitamin A serves in human physiology:

—It is needed to prevent excessive, haphazard bone growth.

—It is required for healthy sperm production.

—It is necessary for good vision.

In this book we are primarily interested in vitamin A's anti-infection properties. According to Wolf, vitamin A is the *anti-infection vitamin* because it's needed to maintain the strength of cell walls so that viruses cannot penetrate. Viruses must enter the cells if they are to survive, for they have no ability to reproduce on their own. Viruses are only able to multiply by taking over the cell's own reproductive mechanism. Instead of producing healthy cells, they invade the cells and produce more viruses. If the process is not stopped eventually, death results.

Usually viruses do not overcome the body. The organism is capable of producing antibodies which can destroy them. It also produces a natural substance, interferon, which in some way, not yet understood, prevents the viruses from utilizing cell reproductive mechanisms. Although the original virus is not destroyed, interferon keeps it from reproducing and spreading the infection.

Now, Dr. Wolf explains that a third means of protection—perhaps most important of all—is also utilized

[23]

by the body. Vitamin A strengthens the cell walls so that viruses are not able to invade the body in the first place.

It is surprising that scientists should have paid so little attention to vitamin A as a weapon against infection in humans. Every researcher on vitamin A knows that if his laboratory animals suffer from a severe deficiency in the nutrient, they become seriously infected and die in a matter of days. According to Wolf, experiments with A-deprived rats in germ-free environments have shown that cell membranes still degenerate, even though the rats do not succumb to infection. But let any germs get at the rats, and the cell walls will immediately be penetrated, and the rats will die.

The same relationship between infection and vitamin A exists in humans, according to several studies. B. M. Kagan reported in the *Journal of Nutrition,* "Children with rheumatic fever have low plasma vitamin A levels. With the onset of increased rheumatic activity the levels drop even further . . . Josephs and Lawrie showed that blood vitamin A levels are reduced in pneumonia and that with convalescence the vitamin A levels rise well above normal. Aron . . . showed that fever, induced by physical means, causes the plasma vitamin A and carotene levels to be lowered and that the degree of lowering is directly related to the duration of fever.

"Moore and Sharman found that liver vitamin A concentrations were low in patients who had abscesses or pneumonia when they died."

Kagan concludes that "the serum vitamin A falls in

[24]

the presence of infection. The fact that the liver vitamin A concentration also becomes low suggests that there is increased demand by other tissues for vitamin A when such infection is present. The only other tissue in which change was found was kidney vitamin A where it was erratically increased. There also appears to be an increase in urine vitamin A. The possibility that it is lost in the urine in a possible detoxification process is suggested."

There is good reason to believe that vitamin A, when applied directly to open wounds, actually hastens the healing process in cases where healing has been retarded due to the use of the steroid drugs, notably cortisone. (Steroids are chemical substances of hormone origin.)

It is precisely this property of vitamin A—the power to fight infection and heal wounds—that makes it important to skin health.

Another form of vitamin A, vitamin A acid, is rapidly becoming a leading therapy in the armamentarium of dermatologists. Skin diseases once considered incurable, even uncontrollable are responding to vitamin A acid.

The *AMA Journal* for March, 1969 carried an article by Drs. Phillip Frost and Gerald D. Weinstein of the Department of Dermatology of the University of Miami School of Medicine dealing with trials they had made of vitamin A acid as therapy for psoriasis and several forms of ichthyosis. In all, 26 patients were treated, all of them having unsightly, distressing and difficult to treat skin disorders.

[25]

Sixteen of 17 patients suffering with Lamellar ichthyosis showed consistent improvement upon treatment with the vitamin A acid ointment. In psoriasis, the doctors found "decreasing scaling and erythema in 24 of 26 patients . . ."

The role vitamin A acid has in treating acne is perhaps its most important one. In June, 1968, at the American Medical Association's 117th annual convention in San Francisco, some of the country's best-known dermatologists responded enthusiastically to a report by James E. Fulton, Jr., M.D., from the University of Pennsylvania School of Medicine, on "Topical Vitamin A Acid in Acne." He presented evidence that the rate of improvement was virtually double in acne patients treated with vitamin A acid, compared with those who used the current treatment of choice benzoyl peroxide.

The B Vitamins

The medical profession has a saying that the dermatologist is the most fortunate of physicians—his patients never die and they never get well. And there is some truth in this. Remarkably little is known about the causes of most skin diseases. The treatments consist largely of remedies that are *believed* to help, but the proportion of failures is so high that the question of whether the successes are due to the self-healing powers of the skin or the medication is seldom resolved.

The problem is that the skin is exposed to so many

threats. Scientists, following the normal pattern of medical investigation, have worked to identify various types of bacteria that might be causing skin diseases, then searched for appropriate antibiotics to destroy them. Boils, for example, are known to be caused by the staphylococcus organism, so efforts have concentrated on treating boils with anti-staph antibiotics. But staph is in the air all around us. Even if an area of the skin were cleansed of these bacteria completely, no doubt they would be found on the skin again in a few hours' time. It is obvious that the real question is how the skin of one individual can fight off these staph organisms without the slightest sign of distress or infection, while in another the same bacteria meet no resistance and are able to penetrate the skin and cause infections.

In other words, a long record of unsuccessful treatment for skin ailments by direct attack on infected areas has made the conclusion almost inescapable: the real problem is one of treating the whole man. We must find and employ methods that will promote general health, including healthy, disease-resistant skin.

At least one prominent dermatologist, Professor Katsu Takenouchi, M.D., professor of dermatology in the School of Medicine of Japan's Chiba University has adopted this approach. In January, 1963, the *Journal of Chiba Medical Society* carried an exciting article by Professor Takenouchi titled "Thiamine Metabolism in the Field of Dermatology." Actually the title is a trifle too narrow in scope, for it was really three vitamins of the B complex with which the dermatologist

[27]

dealt. And here is the first point his laboratory studies were able to establish:

"The presence of inflammation in the skin or the regeneration of the hair in the anagenesis (regeneration) of hair cycle causes a large quantity of glycogen to appear in the prickle cells of the epidermis and the outer root sheath of the hair follicles. Its energy is directed to the repair of inflammation and the regeneration of the skin." And he then goes on to state that contrary to the common belief, the glycogen in the skin does not release its energy without using air but actually has been proven to release it by oxidation.

Such a discovery is of great importance as a demonstration that the skin requires and uses energy in precisely the same way as the internal organs. Glycogen is the storage form of blood sugar or glucose. A healthily functioning liver removes excess glucose from the blood and transforms it into glycogen which it then stores. Whenever the blood sugar level gets too low, the liver releases some glycogen to maintain a normal level. It is thus an enormously important chemical compound within the economy of the human body. And one of the most important single functions of various vitamins of the B complex is that they are indispensable to the metabolic processes by which glucose is converted into glycogen and glycogen is later released and transformed into energy.

If Professor Takenouchi is correct, then the maintenance of a healthy skin and the ability of the skin to fight off infections are dependent on the body's

[28]

having a store of glycogen and being able to use it as required.

Or, to express the same finding in another way, any protracted abnormality of the blood sugar level or any deficiency in even one of the B complex vitamins that are directly concerned with glycogen metabolism can be expected to show up in poor skin health and reduced efficiency in the defense mechanism against infection.

Professor Takenouchi pursued this field of inquiry in the obvious manner. He compared the vitamin B levels in the skins of healthy patients and dermatitis sufferers. With regard to the healthy skin, he found that "Thiamine, riboflavin and pyridoxine have been demonstrated in the skin in relatively large amounts." But he found that 27 per cent of those with various types of dermatoses (skin infections) were deficient or latently deficient in thiamine, 27 per cent equally deficient in riboflavin and 52 per cent deficient in pyridoxine. The small proportion of cases that showed no deficiency in these important B vitamins presumably had either elevated or depressed levels of blood sugar, both of which prevent the proper formation and use of glycogen.

It is clear that to maintain a healthy skin, it is important that the levels of the B complex vitamins be kept high in the system at all times. Professor Takenouchi points out that these water soluble vitamins, even if not used, soon disappear from the skin and must constantly be replaced. He has also computed that only about one per cent of the vitamin B

[29]

we take into our systems is actually channeled to the skin. Thus, to maintain a level of one half a milligram in the skin it is necessary to consume 50 milligrams of thiamine.

Professor Takenouchi has listed the following diseases of the skin directly connected with B vitamin deficiencies in his opinion; eczema, multiple erythema, keratosis, virus disease of the skin, skin tuberculosis, skin syphilis, baldness, and various types of discolorations of the skin.

For some reason Dr. Takenouchi did not investigate for a relationship between B12 and skin health. But the German doctor, H. Grabner, in the *Munich Medical Weekly* (October 31, 1958) described a case history of shingles cured completely in two weeks' time with a combination of vitamin B12 and an antibiotic. Dr. Grabner himself says that he does not know which of the two was responsible for the cure.

Vitamin C

Parents usually resign themselves to the idea that prickly heat, when it develops, must be allowed to run its course. The best they can hope to do is soothe their child's discomfort by applying corn starch (or some other home remedy) to the affected area. Now for the first time a dermatologist from the British Military Hospital in subtropical Singapore has announced a safe and effective cure for this rash—large oral doses of vitamin C. The researcher is Dr. T. C. Hindson, and he made his report in the June 22, 1968 issue of *The Lancet*.

We haven't said nearly all there is to say about the role of vitamins in treating and preventing skin diseases. In fact, you'll find that one or more vitamins have been used successfully in treating any number of skin problems. As we discuss the most common ailments, we will mention the vitamin deficiencies that often lead to them—deficiencies you yourself may be suffering from without realizing it.

But vitamins are only one aspect of the nutrition and skin health story. Some other important ones are discussed in the following chapter.

Chapter IV

The Skin As A Warning Device

The skin is a remarkable barometer which predicts the onset of many illnesses long before any other symptoms appear. It is particularly sensitive to the presence of diseases of the liver and pancreas, according to Dr. Samuel M. Bluefarb and William A. Caro, both of the Department of Dermatology at Northwestern University Medical School in Chicago.

Many of the skin changes are alterations of the pigments. The most common of these is jaundice—the yellowish skin which is often the first sign of liver disease. Jaundice comes from bile, made in excessive amounts, by a sick liver. The bile invades the skin, the mucous membranes and the blood plasma. If the disease that is present is acute hepatitis (a common liver ailment), the jaundice manifests itself rapidly with a strong yellow color. When jaundice occurs in cirrhosis, it is less obvious. The skin might appear pale or gray instead of yellow.

However, cirrhosis often gives other warnings by way of the skin. Itching, another symptom, may come many months before any visible clue. Drs. Bluefarb and Caro describe spider angioma as a sign of cirrhosis. These tumors, usually benign, appear on the face, neck, chest and upper arms. Their apt name comes from their spider-like appearance, characterized by small blood vessels running, like legs, in all directions from the center.

Palmar erythema (red blotches on the palms of the hands) often heralds cirrhosis. Incidentally, this same palmar erythema can be a sign of polyarthritis (arthritis of several joints), endocarditis (inflammation of the valve or lining membrane of the heart), and lung disease.

The abdominal veins, usually all but invisible, may become easy to see and sometimes even bulge above the surface of the abdomen in the presence of cirrhosis. On occasion, they will radiate like spider legs from the navel.

Women suffering from cirrhosis sometimes have skin that is dry and thickened with a rash that produces discolored pimples on the legs and trunk.

In hemochromatosis, a disease of the liver, which gives rise to diabetes, parts of the body turn bluish-gray similar to slate, sometimes bronze or brown. The changes occur most often at the arm pits, the genitalia and adjacent areas, and at the flexion parts of the body such as the insides of the elbows and knees.

Porphria is a liver ailment that affects the metabolism, and can lead to paralysis and mental disturbance; it appears most commonly after injury, such as a bruise, or exposure to the sun. The victim ages visibly, showing a weather-beaten, waxy complexion, with crusted blisters on the face, neck and hands, that leave scars when they heal.

What skin signs point to diseases of the pancreas?—

[33]

a sizeable purple area, like a bruise, below the groin on the left leg or surrounding the navel, might mean a bleeding pancreas; red blotches riddled with a network of tiny blood vessels or threads suggest acute pancreatitis; some victims of pancreatic disease develop tiny fatty nodules beneath the skin, and these may eventually turn into ulcers.

If any of these signs should appear it does not necessarily follow that liver or pancreatic disease is present. It does mean that a thorough checkup is in order.

Chapter V

Are You Photosensitive?

One bright winter morning Betty and John Thompson headed eagerly for the ski slope on a New Hampshire mountainside. It was the first day of their long-awaited second honeymoon. Two days later they had to call it quits. The sunshine was doing terrible things to Betty's skin. Eruptions and yellow-brown patches began to appear not only on her face, but on the exposed parts of her neck as well. Betty—a long-time skier and dedicated sun worshiper—had never experienced a reaction like this.

On the other side of the country, in southern California, a proud mother took her newborn baby for a stroll through the neighborhood on a sunny afternoon. Like Betty on the ski slope, the baby suffered a strong reaction from exposure to the sun—splotchy redness and inflamed tissue wherever his skin was not covered.

Then there was Mr. Henderson, an elderly gentleman recently treated for "anxiety" symptoms. He took a therapeutic walk in the noonday sun of a mild winter day in Chicago. His daughter noticed an eruption on his face and the backs of his hands when he joined the family for dinner that night.

The trouble was identical in each of these cases. A sun-caused dermatitis aggravated by a chemical reaction. Betty had been taking an oral contraceptive, and the estrogen in it had changed her body chemistry, making her "photosensitive" to the rays of the sun. The photosensitizing agent in the baby's case was hexachlorophene in the anti-bacterial soap his mother used to bathe him. Mr. Henderson's reaction was traced to the tranquilizer he was taking—one of the phenothiazines.

Harvard dermatologist Dr. James Kalivas identifies these three compounds as among the many that can induce photosensitivity in susceptible people. His report in the *Journal of the American Medical Association* (September 15, 1969), notes that "cutaneous eruptions more or less confined to light-exposed areas are not uncommon," and he provides a guide for physicians to help them in diagnosis and treatment.

Removal of the offending agent usually ends the problem caused by photosensitization according to the American Medical Association. But the growing number of chemicals in the environment makes the task of finding the culprit harder and harder.

Only lately have physicians recognized the role of chemicals in inducing this super-sensitivity to the sun. As recently as 1952, an article in *The Lancet* stated with some assurance that, while animals are known to become photosensitive through the action of several types of outside agents, in man the only well-known form of photosensitivity is that caused by certain internal diseases. Since these words were published, the proliferation of chemicals in foods and medications

[36]

has become so great that sensitization to sunlight is no longer a rarity.

The distinction between photosensitivity and sensitivity to ordinary sunburn is explained in *Scientific American* (July, 1968), by Farrington Daniels, Jr., Jan C. van der Leun, and Brian E. Johnson. Sunburn is caused by ultraviolet waves. Under certain circumstances, the authors point out "the skin can suffer injury from wave lengths other than ultraviolet, including the radiation in the visible region of the spectrum. In one way or another the skin may become photosensitized, so that substances in the epidermis (outerlayer of the skin) absorb radiation that normally would be harmless, with a consequent formation of free radicals and peroxides that produce cell damage."

The free radicals and peroxides are known to play an important—and perhaps decisive—role in the biochemistry of the aging process, in the opinion of the University of California's Dr. A. L. Tappel *(Geriatrics,* May, 1968.) It is reasonable to assume, then, that a genuine aging of the skin tissue occurs in the case of photosensitized persons.

Dr. Daniels and his co-authors note, in their *Scientific American* article, that many chemicals used in industry, in drugs and in cosmetics, perfumes and antibacterial soaps, are capable of photosensitizing human skin. They believe this hazard "is increasingly a matter of concern in this chemical age."

Fortunately, one such hazard of "this chemical age" —cyclamates—is no longer a problem. There is no way to know how many people suffered unexplained

[37]

rashes, severe burns, and sudden aging of the skin while it was a prime ingredient in numerous low-calorie drinks and foods which were government certified as perfectly safe.

But the ban on cyclamates left literally hundreds of other photosensitizing agents still on the market. They turn up unexpectedly in various drugs and commercial products. Become familiar with the chief culprits, so that you can avoid them when possible. At least you will know what to suspect if you or a member of your family should develop a marked and unusual skin reaction to sunshine.

We have already mentioned three of the chief offenders: birth control pills, tranquilizers and antibacterial soaps. Included in the last are those advertised as deodorant soaps.

Sometimes it is important—in a hospital environment, for example—to use a soap that kills bacteria. But, as a routine "health" measure, it isn't necessary or wise to go around killing all germs. A healthy body can live with all kinds of bacteria; indeed, some bacteria is essential to maintaining good health.

Both the mother who bathes her baby with a bactericidal soap and the teenage boy who uses it to rid his face of acne might bring about the exact reverse of what they are trying to do.

Several types of antibiotics, such as aureomycin and terramycin cause photosensitivity in about 20 per cent of those taking them. Thiazide diuretics also are photosensitizing agents, as are the sulfonamides, whether taken orally or spread on the skin in ointment.

[38]

Antihistamines can cause photosensitization and some antifungal remedies have the same effect.

But quite apart from drugs, photosensitizing chemicals occur in many everyday compounds—insecticides, hair dyes, bleaches and oil-containing cosmetics, fluorescent dyes and tar derivatives.

Certain diseases can also create photosensitization. If you should develop a pronounced sensitivity to sunlight and cannot discover a causative chemical, check with your doctor. Your skin's reaction to the sun could be an early sign of some metabolic disorder or other internal condition that should be treated.

The sun is not always the culprit where photosensitivity is involved.

For a few people whose skins are supersensitive to the invisible ultraviolet rays of the summer sun, fluorescent lighting can spell r-a-s-h. Dr. Ramon M. Fusaro, Minneapolis skin specialist wrote about this in *Minnesota Medicine*. (February, 1969.) Light-sensitivity dermatitis was once easily diagnosed, he says. The doctor simply asked his patient: "Does your dermatitis appear in the spring, get worse in the summer and disappear in the fall?" If the answer was "yes," the doctor knew precisely what he was dealing with. His advice to the patient: protect your skin from sunshine during all but the winter months.

Today, Dr. Fusaro points out, freedom from dermatitis in the colder months of the year "is no longer a significant finding in the diagnosis" of this skin disorder. Because of the ultraviolet rays they receive from

[39]

fluorescent lighting, susceptible persons may develop this form of dermatitis at any season.

Not all fluorescent bulbs are the same in their ultra-violet output, so some cause more severe reaction than others. The ultraviolet rays "may be quantitatively small or very great," depending upon the energy (volt-age) input into the bulb.

The nature of the rash itself is similar to other forms of dermatitis—patchy redness, inflammation, itchiness, possibly the presence of papules (small solid elevations of the skin). But the distribution of the rash provides the best clue. For example, if your fluorescent work lamp is placed on one side of your desk, and your dermatitis is confined to that side of your face and that arm you have reason to suspect the light as the source of your trouble.

You might have an eruption on your face which was caused by the fluorescent fixture at the kitchen sink. Does the dermatitis appear on the portions of your face —forehead and high parts of the cheek—most likely to be reached as you stand there?

If you are sensitive to the ultraviolet rays of fluores-cent lighting, of course you should remove such fix-tures from your house and replace them with incan-descent lights. But lighting in offices and plants cannot always be changed to suit individual employees. Where there is no alternative to fluorescent exposure, Dr. Fusaro suggests sunscreening ointments that might help to keep the dermatitis at a minimum.

Chapter VI

The Myth of the Healthy Tan

One of the most enduring fads of modern times is the "healthy tan." But there is nothing healthy about the "healthy tan." According to the British medical journal, *Lancet,* "Misunderstanding may have arisen from the notion that the tanned outdoor worker, such as the farmer, is leading a healthier life than the pale office clerk. The fact is that the noxious effects of solarization of the white skin far outweigh the beneficial." (May 30, 1970)

Excessive exposure to the sun is a serious threat to health. Millions of workdays a year are lost to American industry because of sunburned absentees. An equal number of days are considered lost due to impaired efficiency because of sunburn. Even more serious, according to Dr. Charles S. Camarron, speaking to the American Cancer Society, "Repeated sunburn is perhaps the most widespread of known causes of cancer."

Dermatologists tell us that constantly repeated exposure to the sun exhausts the skin's healing ability by weakening its pigment and its thickening powers. Persons between the ages of 21 and 50 are said to be particularly susceptible to sunburn, as are pregnant women, presumably due to hormonal changes in the body.

[41]

At the London Institute of Dermatology, in St. John's Hospital for Diseases of the Skin, researchers investigated the now widely accepted conclusion that "the uncovered, sun-exposed skin of man 'ages' more rapidly than covered skin. The most marked effect of such aging is atrophy (drying up) of dermal collagen (the cement that holds the cells together.)"

The ultra-violet rays which are concentrated in sunlight, and in sun lamps, change the texture of the skin to an undesirable quality of toughness and cut down on the vital collagen.

A lesser known side effect of excessive exposure to the sun was discussed by S. William Becker, Jr., M.D., of the Department of Dermatology at the University of Illinois, who has strong reservations about the value of sunlight, especially for light-skinned people. In the (June, 1960) medical publication *G.P.* he points out that after a single moderately-severe sunburn, the blood vessels are affected so adversely that it takes 4 to 15 months for them to return to normal. Sunburning over a period of years dries the skin to the point at which its elasticity is lost. The color darkens and becomes a blotchy brown or yellow.

As we have already suggested, definite skin cancers can and often do develop as the result of too much sun. More than a decade ago Dr. Milton T. Edgerton of Johns Hopkins Hospital, Baltimore, warned that excess exposure to sunshine or sun lamps could cause hundreds of tiny cancers on the face or jaw.

Blondes, particularly blue-eyed blondes, are especially susceptible to skin cancer from excessive sun-

[42]

light as their skins contain little pigment—a part of the skin's protection against too much sun—and they are unable to produce any more of it.

What happens to the skin when it is exposed to the sun? Most of the ultraviolet rays are absorbed by the epidermis. But it may be because some of the ultraviolet rays get through to the dermis, the deep layer of the skin, or because some chemical message is passed from the epidermis, that the minute dermal vessels become dilated and engorged. Other cellular materials, including the elastic fibers of the skin, become heated and disturbed. The malanin pigment, which is found in the deepest layers of the epidermis, begins to migrate upward toward the surface and more of it is produced. Individuals who have sufficient quantities of this pigment, tan. At the same time, the stratum corneum, the outermost layer of cells of the epidermis, becomes thicker.

The evidence indicates that primarily the thickening of the outer layer of the skin, rather than the migration and production of more melanin, protects the skin from further damage upon repeated exposures. The fair skinned Celtic and Nordic peoples, whose skins are most affected by premature aging and cancer formation, have relatively thin skin, whereas blacks and others with darkly pigmented epidermis, generally have a much thicker skin and aging of the skin is remarkably slow in these people.

But repeated, prolonged exposure of the skin to the sun, even for those who tan readily, results in a chemical breakdown of the cells in the underlayer of

[43]

the skin, and chronic, irreversible changes, especially in the elastic fibers. These fibers multiply in number, but become extremely disorganized. The results are atrophy, wrinkling, sagging and drying of the skin. Localized areas of thickening, called keratoses develop and degenerate into basal cell and squamous cell cancers. These changes appear first and are more marked in those areas which have been most exposed to sunlight—the head, neck, hands and forearms.

Dr. Albert Kligman of the Department of Dermatology of the University of Pennsylvania School of Medicine studied the skins of persons from infancy to 90 years old, and found that eighty-seven per cent of the subjects began to show changes in their skin during the second decade of life. By the fifth decade, almost seventy per cent showed the most advanced changes. No white person studied had entirely normal elastic tissue in the skin after 40 years of age.

Dr. Kligman comments, "Most white persons are now obliged to live for more than 70 years. None can escape the cutaneuos ravages of sunlight. . . . I feel strongly that appearance is important to the well-being of the elderly. Good cheer and a robust outlook are difficult to sustain when the dreary ruin of aged skin replaces the fresh skin of the young . . . It is in a way unfortunate that the changes are not visible until decades after they have seriously commenced. The individual has no personal evidence of the insidious decomposition of his skin. Abstract knowledge does not affect behavior unless it is almost unconsciously incorporated by early and pervasive education. A way should be

[44]

found to counteract the manifest attraction of sun-bathing."

The answer, of course, must begin with educating people to the dangers of suntan and the fact that there are no advantages to excessive exposure to the sun's rays. But there must also be a change in social attitudes and values.

Before the turn of the century, when most people worked out of doors, a pale, fair skin was a mark of distinction and a sign of belonging to the leisure (and therefore presumably better) class. But when the majority of productive work moved indoors, a gradual change in attitude took place. Now it was the person with a tanned skin who symbolized leisure and wealth. The viewpoint persists to this day. It will not be easy to turn public opinion back to a sensible and healthful attitude toward solar rays.

If you are required to be out-of-doors during a hot summer afternoon several steps can be taken to safeguard against the sun's rays. The most obvious—because it is the most publicized—is the suntan lotions. The many brands and various types of lotions work in different ways.

The preparations containing zinc oxide or titanium dioxide are opaque and reflect the sun's rays away from your skin; those with benzophenones, absorb the sun's rays before they come in contact with the skin. A third group of chemical agents (the aminobenzoates, salicylates and cinnamates) allows only certain rays of the sun to reach the skin—including the tanning rays.

But commercial suntan lotions are not for everyone.

Some people have bad reactions from a particular chemical on their skins when exposed to the sun's rays. This phenomenon is so common that numerous books and medical journal articles have been written about it—photosensitive contact dermatitis, the scientists call it.

A pharmaceutical tablet that protects against damage from heavy exposure to the sun has been getting wide attention in some circles lately.

Members of the national cricket team of South Africa won't take to the field without it. Competitors in the annual South African canoe races from Pietermaritzburg to Durban are disqualified if they are not using it. A prominent Australian physician reports that several of his patients will avoid all summer outdoor activity if they haven't taken it.

The ingredients of this miraculous tablet: 25,000 milligrams of vitamin A combined with 120 milligrams of calcium carbonate.

E. H. Cluver, M. D. (*South African Medical Journal* 38: 1964), tested the vitamin A-calcium combination on groups of students, with controls, exposed to the same climatic conditions and outdoor sun exposure over a five-year period. He concluded that the tablets do give protection against sun damage, as judged by the development of redness and subsequent peeling. He inferred that the tablets should also protect against sun-caused skin cancers.

Several doctors living in the desert country of central California issued 200 experimental packets of the tablets to volunteers particularly selected because of their sun-sensitivity. (The subjects were either fair and blue-eyed, or redheads.) Half of the packets contained the active vitamin A-calcium substance and the other half contained inert tablets. The patients reported subjectively on their response to sunlight exposure, during the experimental period, compared with their recollection of previous response.

Of the patients actually taking the compound, 63 per cent considered their sun exposure responses "much improved," and 27 per cent said that they were "somewhat improved." None of those on the inert tablets considered that they had increased their resistance to the effects of sunlight, but 25 per cent thought that there was some improvement. Researchers consider this 25 per cent a familiar placebo response.

Ronald Carruthers, M.B., Ch.B., of the Department of Dermatology at Launceston General Hospital in Sydney, Australia calls the positive findings "consistent with those that would be expected if the protection depended . . . on the well-known effect of vitamin A on the skin."

When there is too little vitamin A, the cells on the surface shrivel up and die, and several layers beneath gradually do exactly the same thing. The result is a wrinkly, dry, coarse appearance.

Dr. Carruthers says there are many unexplained features about the action of vitamin A on the epithelial structures. It is interesting, for example, that vitamin A levels in the blood rise after a short exposure to sun, but drop below normal levels if the exposure goes on for a longer period. Yet when G. H. Findley and

[47]

L. W. Van der Nerwe experimented with this phenomenon (*The British Journal of Dermatology,* 77: 1965), they found that even though the vitamin A content in the blood serum fell, there was no compensating rise of vitamin A in the skin. P. Flesch in the *Physiological Review* (50: 1963) explains that ultraviolet rays actually destroy vitamin A. Of course with long exposure more vitamin A is transferred from the blood serum to the skin, where it is destroyed before it has a chance for increased accumulation.

But why add calcium to the anti-sunburn pill? Researchers generally hold that the stored vitamin A cannot be brought from the liver to the skin rapidly enough to counteract the solar shock. Cluver and Politzer state in the *South African Medical Journal* (39: 1965) that an immediate increase in serum vitamin A level is necessary to protect fair-skinned humans. They said the addition of calcium definitely increased the sun-protective effect of vitamin A.

There are other alternatives to commercial suntan preparations and medications. Beauty expert Virginia Castleton Thomas writes about some of them in the June, 1970 issue of *Prevention* Magazine:

"At one point in my travels, I spent some time in the Caribbean. My hostess in Trinidad was an avid gardener, and her flowers were a riot of bloom. Though she spent a great deal of time outdoors, she did not let the sun damage her complexion. She planned her hours to avoid heavy sunlight. Her gardening hours were from early morning until ten o'clock, and then again in late afternoon and early evening.

[48]

"She wore a protective wide brimmed hat and long sleeves at all times outdoors. She carefully maintained her fresh complexion by simply using cocoa butter. Before going outdoors to her work, she gently massaged this greaseless butter onto her face, arms, hands and neck.

"Because the butter melts at body temperature, it seems to sink into the skin. Its application insures against a leathery complexion from moderate exposure to the sun. The cocoa butter also smoothes and softens the textures of skin. So while she was using preventive measures, this island woman was also reaping another beauty dividend . . .

"Wise women, like my friend in the islands, take precautions, for they know it is difficult to restore skin to its original condition after it has been severely damaged . . . Even a young skin can't survive the damaging dryness brought about by sunbathing for long. In time, as oils and moisture are drained from the body, the skin aging process is hastened.

"I recall a neighbor who was startlingly pretty. She had a completely unblemished skin and seemingly, one with no problems. However, she was addicted to the beach. Each year, with her mother and children, she left early in summer for the shore and returned just before school opened in the fall, bronzed like an Aztec princess.

"We all admired her deep tan. Her mother, on the other hand, held no fondness for heavy doses of the sun. She returned each fall little changed in appearance.

[49]

"Once I accepted an invitation to visit them at the shore. It was a pleasant week, centered on the beach. Each morning my neighbor packed a huge basket of food to last until dinner time, and we lay on the beach, or swam. While her mother and I preferred the shade of the beach umbrella, my friend lay prone on the beach, under the direct sun rays. I marvelled at her ability to undergo what would have been torment for me.

"Even before I moved away from her neighborhood, she had begun to age. Her skin did not bounce back during the winter months as it had once done. The darker skin tones began to sit on her face more as a liability than an asset.

"Not too long ago, I saw mother and daughter again, after an absence of some years. Though I recognized the mother, I would not have known the daughter had I met her alone. When I looked at her, I saw a woman, old before her time, with dried, parchment-like skin. There were lines, sagging areas, brown spots, and weariness on her face. This woman had destroyed her once beautiful skin through excess sun exposure."

When selecting a vacation area, or even a new place to live permanently, these sun facts might be helpful in making a healthier choice: The sun's ultraviolet waves are four times greater at the equator than they are in Alaska or upper Sweden. The radiation is one and one-half times greater in the southern than in the northern half of the United States. More radiation comes through at higher altitudes because the air is

[50]

less dense, which is why skiers and mountain climbers get sunburned so easily even in very cold weather.

When sunlight hits the earth's atmosphere, air molecules, dust and water particles scatter the ultraviolet waves, accounting for what is called "sky radiation" which comes at you from all sides. So a beach umbrella provides only partial protection from the sun's rays, even when you are completely in the shade. Still, standing in the shadow of a building protects you from about two-thirds of the harmful intensity of full daylight. The shaded side of the face burns at only half the rate of the exposed side and one-third the rate of the top of the forehead and tops of the ears.

Dry sand reflects about 17 per cent of the burning wave lengths of the sun's rays; but grass only 2.5 per cent. That's one reason it seems to be so much cooler in the country than at the shore, even when the temperatures are similar.

Window glass and glass in automobiles transmits very little erythemal radiation, although the infrared heat waves do come through. Air conditioned cars with closed windows substantially reduce the ultraviolet exposure of those living in hot climates and using such systems.

But the most effective advice when it comes to protection from the sun is still: avoid it as much as possible.

[51]

Chapter VII

Sweat To Save Your Life

Let us say at the outset that sweating is essential to your health. In fact, the function of sweating is one of the most important jobs your skin has.

The body can be compared to an engine with a thermostat. Man produces heat in many ways—by cell activity, muscular activity, digestion of food, and production of hormones. He also picks up heat from the sun.

Whatever the source, the body must protect itself from accumulating too much heat. Under most conditions heat is lost through the skin, through sweat, through the lungs, and through waste. But during exercise, sweat is the key to keeping your cool.

To diminish the effect of body heat, sweat must be permitted to evaporate. It cools the blood close to the surface of the skin, and that blood returns to the body's inner core tissues. At the same time the interior blood carries heat from the inside to be eliminated through evaporation. Circulation also speeds up to make the heat exchange more efficient.

Sudden exposure to high temperatures can cause a reaction called heat exhaustion even though the body sweats properly. The blood rushes to the surface of the body in an effort to carry the core heat to the skin where sweat evaporation can disperse it. As the blood flows to the far-flung capillaries, the blood pressure drops. As the heart becomes less able to maintain blood pressure, there is a slow-down in circulation. The core heat no longer escapes the body and heat exhaustion occurs.

The general signs of heat exhaustion are profuse sweating, a moist skin and a rapid pulse. The victim is usually very uncomfortable and gasps for breath. He may collapse and lose consciousness. Fluids and rest are generally all that is required to bring him back to normal.

Dehydration exhaustion occurs when a person does not drink sufficient liquid to replace body moisture lost while exercising. In very heavy exercise sessions, as much as 8 quarts of water can be sweated away in a 90-minute period. The average water loss in strenuous exercise is around 3 quarts in a 90-minute period. But even this is practically impossible to replenish in 90 minutes. Consequently, there is a decrease in the blood volume and a stimulus is sent to the hypothalamus at the brain. The hypothalamus in turn signals the release of a hormone to slow down the production of urine so more water can be conserved.

If profuse sweating continues and the lost fluid is not replaced, heat stroke follows. Heat stroke is characterized by high temperature and very dry skin. Unless the temperature is reduced promptly, permanent damage to the cells of the brain will occur—and eventually death. For this medical emergency a doctor must be called immediately.

[53]

How does heat stroke develop? It starts with a rising skin temperature, followed by sweating and expansion of the blood vessels. Soon the body's sweating efficiency decreases. As that happens and the blood is no longer cooled adequately, the core temperature rises. When sweating ceases altogether, heat stroke occurs.

There are ways to increase your ability to perform adequately in the heat.

1. During exercise periods replenish fluid loss by sipping water. Some researchers recommend that the water temperature should be around 50° F. The amount of water you drink varies with the heat. Thirst is an excellent guide. When thirsty, drink.

2. If you are eating large amounts of protein foods, you might reduce the amount of protein in your diet somewhat, but be certain to meet minimal needs. Protein creates a greater need for water when digested.

3. Sweating uses up important minerals—sodium chloride (salt) and potassium. Both are very important and must continually be replaced. Yet, salt tablets are recognized by some authorities as dangerous.

The answer is to eat some foods that are naturally high in salt and potassium. Celery, sea foods, ham, raisins and spinach are all salty. Spinach is also rich in potassium, as are prunes, almonds and peanuts, bananas and such leafy vegetables as broccoli and cauliflower. With the possible exception of active, professional athletes, diets heavy in these foods will provide the necessary salt and potassium for most people.

4. Air-conditioning can play havoc with your

body's ability to adjust to heat. Sitting in an air-conditioned house, office, or car all day and then going out to play golf for four hours in 90° temperature is quite dangerous. The shock is simply too great for the body to overcome.

5. Develop a better fitness level. Research studies have shown that the more fit a person is, the more rapidly he will become acclimatized and the more efficient his sweating mechanism will be. And the less body salt he will lose during exercise.

6. Never exercise when the relative humidity exceeds 97 percent. Air that is virtually saturated with water will not be able to take up adequate amounts of water from the body surface. In that situation, the body will not cool adequately and body temperature can rise alarmingly.

7. Follow the Wet Bulb Temperature Guide. This guide has been established to give you an idea of when and how much to exercise.

*Wet Bulb Temperature Guide

Under 60° F	No precautions necessary
61-65° F	Be alert for any unusual signs, especially if prone to great water loss
66-70° F	Take small amounts of water while exercising

*(Adapted from R. J. Murphy & W. F. Ashe, *Journal of American Medical Assocaition* 194: 180, 1965.)

[55]

71-75° F   Practice above precautions and provide rest periods every 30 minutes

76° F and up   Practice above precautions and wear shorts or do not exercise at all

For health, it is necessary to sweat. But socially, there is a taboo against body odor from perspiration.

There is nothing wrong with neutralizing perspiration odors as long as the methods are not injurious to health. But look at the commercial deodorants that are urged upon us through every medium of advertising, and what do you find? By the best and most expert professional evaluation obtainable, every one of them is somewhat toxic. Sometimes deodorants are combined with antiperspirants, which are chemicals that attempt to prevent odors by sealing up the pores so that perspiration is slowed or stopped in areas where it is normally profuse, such as the armpits. This practice of inhibiting or preventing perspiration is dangerous both in its intent and because of the toxic nature of the materials used.

The monumental encyclopedia of toxicity information that is compiled and periodically updated, *Clinical Toxicology of Commercial Products,* lists the ingredients of commercial products in common use and rates their known degree of toxicity on a scale from 1 to 6. Only the 1 rating indicates a lack of ill effects in any degree at all. Examine the formulations of commercial deodorants, and you find that most of them have a toxicity rating of either 2 or 3. This does not mean that they will kill you. But it does mean that they can evoke some unhealthy reaction and might harm some of their users while deodorizing them.

Stick deodorants ordinarily contain *oxquinoline sulfate* which is a moderately toxic chemical known as a stimulant of the central nervous system. *Sodium hydroxide* turns up in some stick deodorants and is nothing other than caustic soda, which even in small quantities can easily burn a delicate skin.

Deodorants may also contain *benzoic acid,* which has been known to cause convulsions and death in a baby and *chloral hydrate,* otherwise known as the Mickey Finn, will cause unconsciousness and sometimes death if a few drops are swallowed. It is a corrosive agent.

We could go on but long lists of ingredients are tedious, the point is that most commercial deodorants contain some toxic material.

The net result is that the user risks skin burns, drying out precious skin oils, blackheads, and much worse if the chemicals are absorbed through the skin.

And all this is true of men's and women's lotions.

Women have been trying to smell like flowers for hundreds of years, but only recently the cosmetics industry began pushing the idea that men should smell like pine trees, perfumed leather, or like their wives. Men have been buying the new colognes and aftershave lotions with the result that the incidence of perfume dermatitis in men has been rising. Ernst Epstein, M.D., a dermatologist in San Mateo, California, has treated increasing numbers of male patients suffering from itching, eczematous inflammations of the skin of the face, neck, ears, eyelids and hands.

Using the patients' own perfumes, Dr. Epstein established that the men had allergic reactions to perfumes. The incidence of perfume dermatitis in men is likely to go up, says Epstein, as a result of the intensive advertising campaigns that are making such preparations increasingly popular.

Careful body hygiene can do much to prevent odor offense to others. Try to depend on showers and bathing to eliminate body odors. Dust cornstarch on after a bath. If you must use a deodorant, use it as little as possible. Do not use any odor-combating substance in the presence of skin disease, and don't use any of these substances immediately after a bath when all the pores are open.

Deodorants containing aluminum compounds are especially irritating. Try to avoid these. If you intend to use a deodorant or antiperspirant on an area that you have shaved (such as the underarms) avoid application immediately after shaving, since the skin is raw and irritation is more likely at this time.

If you are bothered by body odors to the extent that you definitely intend to use a deodorant, by all means, avoid the antiperspirant type. Sweating can save your life.

Chapter VIII

The Mystery Rashes

Probably the most common skin ailments of all are those that, at first glance, seem to be without cause. They are the rashes on the feet, the blotches on the back or face, the red, blistering hands. They are the purple spots, the red welts, the dry, cracked patches. And, for the life of us, we cannot figure out where they came from.

Because they are so common, medical science has been spending a good deal of time and money investigating these mystery skin diseases, so that today, we have a great deal of helpful information about their causes and treatments.

For example, we know that most of these ailments are allergies. They can be caused by the clothes you wear or the cosmetics or soap you use (contact dermatitis), the medication you take, pollution in the air you breathe, the lighting in your home and a host of other factors. Sometimes the allergy shows up only under exposure to the ultraviolet rays of the sun. This phenomenon is called "photosensitivity."

The American Dermatological Association has no exact statistics on the number of Americans suffering from skin allergies. However, chances are good that if you are suffering a mysterious skin problem, it is due to an allergy. Here are several of the most common of these, their causes and treatments:

Shoes

When the young woman first came to Dr. Ernst Epstein's office in San Mateo, California, she could hardly walk. Her feet were swollen and inflamed—the skin was cracked and scaly.

She had been suffering with this problem for five years. The disease had steadily progressed. Four dermatologists as well as her own physician had been consulted, and no two of their diagnoses agreed. None of the prescribed treatments had helped.

A 16-year old track star visited Dr. Epstein with a similar complaint. Itching and stinging red blotches covered every inch of his feet and ankles. Almost unbearable irritation developed between his toes. The doctors were baffled.

To most doctors, these cases would represent rare and puzzling "mystery diseases." But to Dr. Epstein, who has seen at least 40 similar cases in the last few years, there was a simple explanation: dermatitis from shoes. Speaking at the 117th Annual Medical Convention in San Francisco in June, 1968, Epstein told physicians from all over the country, "Shoe contact dermatitis is far from rare. Yet it is often overlooked by doctors, and scarcely ever mentioned in medical texts."

Before 1940, shoe contact dermatits was, in fact, virtually unheard of. But today, there are hundreds of cases documented in medical literature. It is impossible to estimate, of course, how many thousands more have gone undiagnosed.

Usually the irritation centers around the large toe, but it can spread between all the toes. It is frequently mistaken for athlete's foot or another fungus growth, but fungicide ointments and other preparations of that kind are ineffective in treating it. Sometimes it is mistaken for eczema. The disease can spread to the hand, and in 1 out of every 8 of Epstein's patients, it did.

One unmistakable sign is a rash that exactly matches the skin's point of contact with the shoe—for example, the strap of a woman's shoe. When it occurs, those particular shoes should be discarded at once.

When the young woman mentioned before first visited Epstein, she was typical of those suffering with shoe contact dermatitis. Epstein, who had been working with similarly afflicted patients for many years, immediately began testing for allergic reactions to some of the chemicals used in shoe making. Top priority was given to testing for reactions to the rubber additives. (They are responsible for 18 of every 20 cases of shoe dermatitis.) A patch test for rubber additives caused a positive reaction in the young woman, and within a few days the five years of foot misery were ended. It was found that two out of three pairs of shoes the woman wore frequently contained the additives to which she was allergic. Shoes free of them were ordered, and the woman has been without symptoms since.

Most rubber-allergic people react because of "accelerators" or "anti-oxidants," such as mercaptobenzthiazole or tetramethylthiuram sulphide. These two chemicals are used very commonly in rubber manufacturing. Rubber glues that are used to hold shoes together also cause trouble for a number of people.

The rubber chemicals were also responsible for the problems suffered by the young athlete. Epstein's investigation showed that the boy wore sneakers with rubber padding and the padding contained the additives that triggered the dermatitis. When the boy shifted to other footwear, his condition improved.

Since the shoe's rubber-based adhesive is so often the allergen that produces shoe dermatitis, suspected victims should look for clues to rubber sensitivity in other areas of the body that have contact with rubber—elastic waistbands, for example. Among Dr. Epstein's patients, several had waist dermatitis from underwear; a rubber garter strap had caused a rash on the thigh of one woman, and another had had dermatitis induced by a rubber bathing cap.

Rubber additives are not the only cause of shoe contact dermatitis. In fact, the very first case reported in the medical literature (*Archives of Dermatology and Syphilology,* 19, 175, 1929) was caused by an ingredient in the leather of the shoe.

When more than 100 British sailors had to be sent home from the tropics a few years ago, because they became invalids from severe dermatitis of the foot, the culprit turned out to be leather sandals. (*British Journal of Dermatology,* 78, 617, 1966). The chemical that usually causes the trouble in leather is potassium dichromate, a substance commonly used in the tan-

[62]

ning process. Small particles of chrome actually become fixed into the leather, and when the foot sweats, they are released. When they come into contact with the foot of a person who is allergic to them, the chrome particles can cause a severe reaction in the skin. Sometimes doctors, when taking skin samples, can actually detect the chrome particles in the tissue.

The young woman and the high school athlete who consulted Dr. Epstein were both very lucky. Although they suffered from a most unpleasant, sometimes painful disease, they were allergic to only one substance—rubber additives. And the British sailors were affected only by the chrome used in the tanning process. Once the allergen was identified, the cure was simple: a new pair of shoes minus the allergen.

But for many, the whole picture is much more complex. In the past, a person allergic to chrome-tanned leather shoes merely switched to vegetable-tanned ones. But, now we read (*The Lancet,* February 11, 1967), that, vegetable-tanned leather (especially East Indian) is a much commoner cause of allergy than the chrome-tanned variety. And the nature of the allergen in vegetable-tanned leather is undetermined.

And that is only the beginning. A hyper-allergic individual must also be careful of the material used for making the eyelets of the shoe. Nickel is often used for that purpose—and researchers report that nickel causes shoe contact dermatitis in some people.

When victims of shoe dermatitis discovered a company in Brockton, Massachusetts that made a "non-allergenic" shoe, they thought they had found the solu-

[63]

tion to all their problems. Then a New Orleans physician reported that a number of his patients had reacted to paraphenylenediamine, a dye found in the Brockton shoes.

Epstein suggested that people suffering from multiple shoe allergies, might consider lining their shoes with Saran Wrap or plastic lining. But, again, some people are allergic to the plastic.

It is not easy to determine from the salesman at a shoe store whether or not such-and-such an allergen is present in the finished article, because shoe companies are reluctant to divulge what additives they use in making their shoes. However efforts are being made to require the manufacturer to state, for every type of shoe, whether the leather is full-chrome, semi-chrome or vegetable-tanned, and whether any of the well-known sensitizers are present in the rubber cement.

But it is not the kind of thing in which the public can simply demand action. Physicians have a responsibility. As Epstein said, "Patients with shoe dermatitis will continue to be overlooked unless doctors take this problem seriously." Meanwhile if shoe contact dermatitis is your problem, try switching to shoes that contain no rubber and are not glued together. If your trouble persists, it may be necessary to have your shoes custom made, of non-allergic materials.

Clothes

As long ago as October, 1957, the *Journal of the American Medical Association* reported that drip-dry fabrics, commonly used for women's dresses and men's shirts, and underwear of both sexes, get their crease-resisting qualities by adding formalin or formaldehyde to the textiles. The A.M.A. Journal article pleaded with manufacturers of such fabrics to list the added chemicals on the labels, so that those with related allergies might be warned. To the best of our knowledge, no American manufacturer has done it yet.

Mr. D., a man of 52, complained to his doctor that for the past three years he had suffered intermittently from red, scaly, oozing and itchy skin at the backs of his knees and at the inside areas of his thighs. A series of tests revealed an allergy to formaldehyde. He was told to stop wearing durable press trousers, and, when he did, his trouble disappeared.

Urea formaldehyde, a type of resin used to add convenience features in the finishing of fabrics, has long presented problems to many who wear drip-dry and permanent press clothing. However, since 1964 when no-iron slacks were first delivered to retail stores, millions of dollars have been spent to produce no-press shorts, skirts, suits, dresses, shirts and pants. Experts estimate that at least 80 percent of all men's slacks and dress shirts and 70 percent of all sport shirts are now in the durable press (dp) category. The dp industry is still growing; the textile industry in general has never enjoyed such a boom. Yet, the dp process contains some inherent health hazards for all who would like to wear this clothing. Let's examine this procedure:

The factory making durable press fabric blends natural fiber cotton with a synthetic fiber such as nylon

[65]

or polyester. Then they impregnate this fiber blend with a finishing compound (the resin), which causes the fibers to develop a "memory" of their original form and shape. Using the "deferred cure," they let this sensitized fabric dry at room temperature.

The clothing maker will then cut and sew the material into the desired garment, press in pleats and creases, press out wrinkles. He cures the garment by baking it in an oven of 325 to 350 degrees for 15 to 19 minutes. In this final step the resin links the synthetic and natural fibers in such a way that no more wrinkles can be put in and no creases can be removed.

On the surface, durable press garments seem to be a great boon. But there are many people—perhaps millions—who are allergic to urea formaldehyde resins. Some of them never discover it, though they suffer from the symptoms. And the allergies get worse if they are continually restimulated. Unfortunately, the allergen, urea formaldehyde, is becoming harder and harder to avoid.

E. E. O'Quinn, M.D. and C. B. Kennedy, M.D., writing in the *American Medical Association Journal* (November 8, 1965) attributed the skin disorders, which appear after wearing certain clothing, to the fiber, "soaps or detergents carried on the material, or to dyes, rubber, formaldehyde or other textile-finishing compounds." The early stages of irritation consists of itching, reddening and pimples. As the ailment becomes more chronic, scaling and lesions can appear. Women seem to be more sensitive to dp than men are.

[66]

Even thorough laundering does not eliminate the possibility of formaldehyde coming into contact with the skin. O'Quinn and Kennedy noted that irritation is most likely in sweat gland areas, since heat and moisture tend to encourage the release of the free formaldehyde.

"Scotchguard" is another chemical used in fabrics which has come under fire for causing skin problems. When it was introduced several years ago, it quickly became a favorite for upholstery materials as well as wearing apparel. Customers were intrigued with the possibility of easily wiping up accidental spills that would ordinarily have led to serious stains in fabrics. The "Scotchguard" protection on fabric has become widely prevalent, but buyers are learning that the price of such protection might be serious personal discomfort for those allergic to this chemical compound.

Soaps

The value of soap and baths for removing skin bacteria was put to the test some years ago and the report appeared in *The Lancet*. It said that the effect of bathing, in respect to shedding bacteria from the skin of subjects, actually tended to increase the bacterial fallout for a short time. Baths, it was suggested, only loosen particles of skin.

Dr. Ralph C. Richards, University of Utah surgery professor, said, in the November, 1968 *University of Utah Review,* the "proportion of bacteria removed

[67]

from the body by bathing is almost insignificant, probably no more than seven percent."

"A bath a day is not only unnecessary but often harmful," adds Dr. Ralph V. Platou, a New Orleans pediatrician. Speaking at the Tennessee Pediatric Society in September of 1965, he went on to say, "Most of us are bathed too much. Today's stronger soaps can remove many of the natural skin secretions which are beneficial. We should be bathed where we are dirty and only when needed. Otherwise our skin should be left alone."

Writing in *The New Scientist,* Dr. F. Ray Bettey (a British dermatologist) accuses soaps made the traditional way, from caustic alkalies and fats, of not only removing grease and dirt, but of penetrating the skin's protective layers and leaching out the skin's protective emulsion, frequently causing chapping or more severe inflammation. Also, soaps are usually alkaline and therefore reduce the acidity on which the skin relies to help kill bacteria.

This is probably the most important single reason for reducing the use of soap as much as possible.

A. L. Hudson, M.D., of Toronto, Canada, writing in the *Canadian Medical Association Journal,* discusses the effect of soaps and detergents as well as different drugs, shampoos and ointment on the skin. We have somehow come to think of alkalinity as something to be highly desired. But when speaking of the skin, it is well to remember that alkalinity is not normal.

According to Dr. Hudson, in parts of the body where a great deal of perspiration is excreted, the acidity is greater. And, naturally, in hot weather this pH goes even lower, for then there is more perspiration. This normally acid condition of the skin is spoken of as "the acid mantle." If the acid condition of the skin is maintained, the chances for development of contact dermatitis are lessened, the skin is most susceptible in the alkaline state.

Tests have shown that a skin area with a normal pH of four, shows a pH of seven one minute after it is washed with soap and it may take 70 minutes for the skin to return to its normal pH. With some soaps, this increased alkalinity may persist for as long as 3½ hours. We should keep in mind that when we talk of alkalinity in connection with soap, we mean all soap, because alkali is set free in water as soon as soap is put into it and the alkalinity of the solution may rise to as high as 10 or 11.

Variations in normal skin acidity occur according to: the character and quantity of perspiration, the prevention of evaporation of this perspiration, the amount of secretion of the oily glands of the skin which becomes alkaline as it is evaporating. So the acidity of the skin and, to a certain extent, the health of the skin, depend on the composition of sweat and how much of it is left unevaporated on the skin. Other conditions aside from washing with soap make the skin alkaline— dust, disintegrated sweat glands, tuberculosis, seborrhea, psoriasis, and several other skin diseases. When there are certain kinds of disorders present in the skin, this change to alkalinity is more marked and more prolonged in the diseased area and the skin around it.

[69]

It seems obvious that medicines, ointments or soaps applied to any part of the body where the alkalinity is already high should be acid if possible. This is especially true with fungus growths, such as cause athlete's foot. Any medication used here should make the skin more, not less, acid. Of course, soap on athlete's foot is bound to increase the alkalinity still further and make the condition worse.

If your hands, feet and legs suffer from the cold weather (and what housewife doesn't have trouble with rough, painful hands in winter?) you would do well to take every precaution against exposure to soaps and detergents. Too many of us are likely to dismiss rough winter hands as "a bad case of chapping" and rub on some lotion which we hope will make them smooth again. Alkaline soaps and detergents, as we have seen, produce a definite unhealthy state of skin by the chemical action, and many kinds of disorders may result. Now lined rubber gloves with ridged fingers are available—efficient and easy to put on and remove. Every one should wear them when working with soap and water.

Detergents

In the days before detergents, we used to speak of the curse of "dishpan hands." Now, with the onslaught of the "miracle" cleaners, our hands have not only that tell-tale roughness, but cases of real skin disease are cropping up which can definitely be traced to constant contact wth the new "grease cutters."

[70]

Though the advertisers claim that the new soapless detergents are the joy of the housewife—time-savers that eliminate unnecessary scrubbing, labor-savers that eliminate rinsing, beautifiers that make clothes dazzle, that make dishes fairly sparkle, there is, of course, no mention of the possible loss of time, beauty, and even health that results from their bad effects on the hands.

Why this harsh talk about detergents? Do they really have such a bad effect on our hands? There is no question about it, detergents do dry up the skin and cause irritation.

The standard test two well-known detergent-makers used to demonstrate the effectiveness of their products proves the point. The manufacturers made up a detergent solution and floated a live duck on the surface. A duck has a small gland in the top part of his back that secretes oil, which keeps his feathers oily enough so that he can stay afloat in water. When placed on the detergent much of the duck's buoyancy was lost and he struggled to keep afloat. Not very nice for the duck. But it shows how the natural oils are broken down. So how about your hands?

Detergents are substances much like soap, but their molecules are arranged differently. This is what gives them their miraculous cleansing power. Detergents are made from petroleum or coal. They are coal tar products which are, one by one, being proved to be highly toxic to living organisms.

One of the most frequent advertising claims of all detergents is their ability to penetrate and cling to the

[71]

surface of whatever they are used on. After they have dissolved the dirt and grease, they needn't be rinsed off. *"Glasses sparkle without rinsing or wiping."* Just so. The detergent stays on—and you drink or eat a bit of it with every meal, to say nothing of the quantities your hands absorb washing dishes, plus laundry, plus any number of other detergent-and-water jobs.

But we are not concerned primarily with the effects detergents have on the entire body—just the skin. When detergents were new, almost twenty years ago, Dr. Martin F. Engmen, Jr. wrote in the *American Practitioner and Digest of Treatment* for June, 1954, "Since the advent of the new soapless detergents, the number of cases of housewives' eczema has increased many times." He admitted that the cause cannot be given simply, but "housewives eczema of the hands is the most prevalent industrial skin disease"—considering housewifery as the largest industry in the world.

Time Magazine once named skin eruptions on the hands as "responsible for much misery, and for a big share of a dermatologist's practice nowadays . . ." An Eczema-like eruption of the hands is often caused by the defatting and drying effects of soap and detergents used in dish washing, especially during cold weather.

The solution is not easy. When the main aim of washing appears to be to get it over with in the best, quickest, and easiest fashion, it is hard not to use the product that achieves this end. But, in spite of what

[72]

may seem like inconveniences, skin specialists, advise cutting out detergents.

Sensitizers By The Score

We have hardly scraped the surface in discussing the substances in our environment which can lead to contact dermatitis. These substances, almost without exception are man-made. In effect, contact dermatitis is just anoher disease of civilization.

This fact is nowhere better illustrated than in our cities, where air pollution is rampant.

Marble, concrete and granite will begin to disintegrate after a few years of steady exposure to sulfur dioxide pollution in the air; tough nylon stockings literally fall apart when certain chemical concentrations are high in the atmosphere. If stone and nylon can't take it, do you wonder that human skin problems from air pollution are becoming commonplace? Layers of air-borne soot and dust that coat the skin of city dwellers are bound to interfere with its regular texture and function.

Irwin I. Lubowe, M.D., F.A.C.A., writing in *General Practice* (May, 1964) stated flatly: "The possible relationship of air pollutants and skin health cannot be dismissed without serious consideration . . . There is also an increase in collagen diseases which may be associated with autoimmunization reactions related to air pollution."

Doctors were stumped recently when a 51-year-old man presented himself for diagnosis of a mysterious

[73]

skin disease of his hands. He said it all began when he took up golf several years before, and though certain medications seemed to bring relief, the itching and skin eruptions only disappeared entirely at the end of the golf season. Each year it got worse, eventually involving his arms, legs, neck, face and wrists. The disease grew worse the day after the greens were sprayed. The patient noted that his right hand, the one used to pick up the ball, was most severely involved.

Doctors investigated the spray used by the golf course. A few milligrams brought into contact with the patient's skin produced large eczematous reactions coupled with a generalized flare-up. The patient was extremely sensitive to the thiram compound in the fungicide used at the golf course.

Thiram is one of the primary causes of rubber sensitivity, according to Walter B. Shelley, M.D., writing in the *Journal of the American Medical Association* (May 4, 1964). The thiram-sensitive individual must avoid all types of rubber products including art-gum erasers, bunion pads, eyelash curlers, mattresses, rubber gloves, shoes, adhesives, dentures, bathing caps, headrests, garters, toys and even girdles.

Thirty years ago thiram was introduced as a powerful fungicide, and soon it was being dusted and sprayed on farms, lawns and golf courses. But that was only the beginning. Now thiram is used to treat fabrics and wood. Seeds, plants, fruits, vegetables, nuts and mushrooms also get the thiram treatment to prevent fungus. In 1956 a survey showed that thiram also acts as a sun-screening agent. Several thiram-containing sun-tan sprays appeared after that and, of course, contact dermatitis turned up in some of the users.

It is true, the normal skin has built-in defenses against the invasion of some harmful foreign elements. There are two important barriers, the horny layer of epidermis and the oily secretion of the sebaceous glands. But many substances do get through these defenses and reach the living cells beneath the skin in sufficient quantities to cause sensitivity that shows up in the form of itchy or painful blistering and scabbing.

Eczema—often called the asthma of the skin—is an itchy, red skin rash that has also been found related to air pollution in some cases.

"An Effect of Continued Exposure to Air Pollution on Incidence of Chronic Childhood Disease" by Harry A. Sultz, M.D., and associates presented at the November 1969 meeting of the American Public Health Association studied the incidence of both asthma *and eczema* in children under 16 years of age in the Buffalo, New York, area. All of the cases in the study were severe enough to warrant hospitalization. The results of the study point conclusively to air pollution levels (measured by suspended particles) as the causative factor.

In the nine-year period from 1961-1969, the researchers studied 617 hospitalized cases of acute asthma and another 165 hospitalized cases of eczema. Here is what the investigators found: Percentage wise, the asthma cases climbed consistently from 86 percent at the lowest air pollution level to 114 percent at the highest. With eczema, the average annual incidence

[75]

rate of hospitalized cases rose as much as four times due to highly polluted air.

So, ezcema joins the already long list of diseases linked to air pollution. Though a parent can protect his child from eating foods to which he is allergic, how can he prevent the child from breathing the impure air? Though he can clean his home of dust and hydrocarbons, how can he clear his house of poluted air? The answer is that short of supplying his child with a miniature gas mask to wear every day (and even that won't really allay the insidious effects of air pollution) he can't.

In addition to the air out of doors there are unsuspected enemies to your skin in the house. Those no-iron, long-wearing curtains made of glass fiber, for example, can affect the skin, according to Canadian dermatologist Dr. Benjamin K. Fisher. He said that microscopic glass fibers can become imbedded in the rest of the family laundry in the washing machine and cause painful skin irritation in the wearers. The *Denver Post* (November 20, 1968) reported that many skin specialists are encountering patients with dermatitis caused by strands of glass fibers. Dr. Fisher urges that glass fiber material be labeled for laundering separately from other fabrics.

And who would ever suspect that the menthol used in cigarettes, candy and cough drops can cause skin problems? When an 18-year old girl presented herself before E. M. McGowan, M.D., the rash all over her body was obvious. After the usual allergy tests proved fruitless, he asked about her menthol consumption.

[76]

She admitted smoking menthol cigarettes, eating menthol-flavored candy, using menthol cough drops, and brushing her teeth with mint-flavored tooth paste. Dr. McGowan told her to eliminate all menthol products, and her rash disappeared.

In his article in the *Archives of Dermatology* (May, 1967) McGowan suggested that some men who put up with a stubborn rash on their faces might find that it is caused by the "cool" mentholated shaving cream or lotion they use. Mysterious rashes might be tracked down more readily if physicians questioned patients carefully about the menthol products they use.

Even a beloved pet can be an enemy to your skin. Dogs infected with scabies, a skin disease, can pass on their affliction to humans, says an Indianapolis, Ind., physician who studied children infected by pet puppies. Dr. A. L. Norins observes that dog-caused scabies should be suspected if several members of the family contract dermatitis shortly after a new pet is brought into the home.

An increasing number of allergic dermatitis cases in adolescent girls has been attribtued to the manner in which ears are pierced and earrings worn. The only way to avoid this condition, say dermatologists, is to keep the channels open with high quality gold or silver wires or black silk thread. Earrings should not be worn until the channels have healed, and those with an allergic reaction to nickel should take care to avoid posts made with that metal.

By now you can see that any number of seemingly harmless substances in your environment (from the air

[77]

you breathe to the shoes you wear) can be the cause of those mysterious rashes. And that is just the beginning. There are many more seemingly harmless substances that you come into contact with every day that can pose serious threats. Some of them are drugs. Others are cosmetics you might use to improve your skin. Ordinarily they may be helpful, or at least do you no harm. But for many people who have a peculiar sensitivity, some of the chemicals in them can cause unsightly and painful reactions when the user comes into contact with the ultraviolet rays of the sun. We discuss this problem in detail in another chapter.

Chapter IX

Prickly Heat

Prickly heat is a common summertime ailment. In temperate climates such as ours, babies suffer from it more frequently than adults—but the disease is not rare in adults, and often occurs on the inside of the thighs at the groin.

The rash develops very quickly as a result of excessive sweating, and can occur wherever such sweating takes place. If one side of a baby's face is pressed against the pillow or a nurse's uniform for any length of time, prickly heat can be expected. If a diaper is tight and warm enough to cause profuse sweating, the rash will probably develop. Tiny, slightly inflamed pimples develop on the skin surface accompanied by a tingling and itching sensation. Within a few days the pimples become blisters containing a milky substance. They disappear quite soon, leaving tiny scabs which scale off.

But sometimes, especially in children, the itching becomes unbearable. The youngsters scratch until an infection develops and, with it, a much more serious problem. No adequate treatment had been available before now.

Dr. Hindson, writing in *The Lancet,* gives convincing evidence that vitamin C can effectively treat prickly heat. He writes, "Of 15 children given ascorbic acid for two weeks, 14 improved. . ."

Hindson stumbled across this powerful treatment by a stroke of luck. An Australian Air Force officer came to his office one day suffering from a severe case of prickly heat (technically known as malaria rubra papulosa). The patient told Hindson that he had had the rash for a year, and that all the forms of therapy he tried had been ineffective.

As Hindson continued to interview the officer, the Australian remembered that the rash had suddenly disappeared for a short time while he was taking vitamin C to treat a cold.

"I put him on ascorbic acid, one gram daily as the sole treatment, and when reexamined ten days later his groin was normal," writes Hindson.

The dermatologist felt that he was on to something important. He chose five children—patients of his—who suffered from recurrent, severe prickly heat. Each was given doses of vitamin C. The result: no further attacks of prickly heat occurred while they were taking the vitamin.

But such evidence alone does not win the support of the medical community. Perhaps these cases were rare coincidence. Perhaps other factors were involved. More adequate criteria were needed if Hindson's theory was to gain a hearing by other physicians. "Subsequently I carried out a double-blind trial of ascorbic acid in the treatment of 30 cases of prickly heat," Hindson writes.

The criterion Hindson established for selecting his 30 cases was that all patients should have suffered continuously from prickly heat for a period of eight weeks, immediately before his initial interview with them. The children were divided into two equal groups. Half were given vitamin C, and half a placebo (a tablet or liquid which looks like the medication but actually has no effect whatever). Hindson guarded against unconsciously influencing the patients by having the pharmacist select each group without Hindson's knowledge.

Before the experiment was begun, Hindson had to decide how much vitamin C should be administered daily. He took as his guide the amount that had been used by the Australian Air Force officer—one gram daily for a person weighing 150 pounds. (A gram is equivalent to 1000 milligrams.)

Some children were too young to take the tablets, so Hindson instructed parents to crush them thoroughly and mix them in with food. After two weeks, he tabulated the results.

Two of the 15 on the placebo showed no sign of the rash. Ten on the vitamin C showed no sign. Whereas 2 more on the placebo showed considerable signs of improvement, 4 on the vitamin showed similar signs. On the placebo, 9 showed no change and 2 grew worse. Of those taking the vitamin, only one showed no change, and none was worse.

Hindson then gave the vitamin to the 15 patients who had been on the placebo. After two weeks, 6 had no sign of prickly heat, and 5 had considerably improved.

Hindson isn't sure why the vitamin works. Past research suggests that prickly heat occurs when the

[81]

sweat glands in a particular area of the body stop working. These glands usually stop functioning because of fatigue. They have been overtaxed and overworked for too long and just take a vacation. That is why prickly heat and similar irritations of the groin are common in hot climates where the sweat glands are continually taxed.

While admitting that the exact mechanism by which vitamin C prevents prickly heat has not been established, Dr. Hindson says that vitamin C acts as a hydrogenion carrier for certain enzyme systems which relate to the sweat glands. When the sweat glands are overtaxed, perhaps a shortage of the vitamin develops and the enzyme does not function adequately.

Another possibility Hindson suggests is that "the vitamin in large doses might take over the action of, or replenish some essential but fatigued enzyme system— such as the succinic-dehydrogenase system—which Dodson (1958) showed was the first to disappear on excess sweating. . ."

Hindson points out that vitamin C levels have never been determined in sweat collected from individuals on high ascorbic-acid intake. But what this researcher has proven rather conclusively is that, "Ascorbic acid, when given in high doses, is effective in the treatment and prevention of prickly heat."

Chapter X

Burns

Serious burns are usually classed as second, third and fourth degree burns. The higher the degree, the greater the depth and severity of the burn. Most of us have experienced a first degree burn, the type in which the skin becomes reddened and irritated, but does not blister or break. An ordinary sunburn is considered a first degree burn. In second degree burns there is partial destruction of the skin, but it is not lifeless. Blistering is the most common indication of a second degree burn. In third or fourth degree burns, the skin has been destroyed through its full thickness, sometimes through underlying tissues down to the bone. It is dry and firm, leathery to the touch. A charred-appearing skin is the mark of a fourth degree burn.

Techniques used in the treatment of burns have improved in recent years and have increased the chances of survival considerably. Fifteen years ago, recovery from burns which covered one-third, or more, of the body was uncommon. Today, even if one should sustain serious burns that cover as much as half of the body area, the possibility of recovery is strong.

There are three main phases in the clinical history of serious burns. The first is a period of shock, in which there are pronounced shifts in body fluids and electrolytes in the burned area, a loss of plasma and protein, and possible damage to various organs, as well as the involved tissue. This period, which is in force from the moment the burn is incurred, is followed by a critical second period during which secondary anemia usually develops and infection of the injured area is likely. This stage lasts for about 10 days to two weeks, and is followed by the final period of healing and repair.

One often sees the term "shock" used in connection with severe burns. Shock is a condition in which the blood pressure is reduced to a point of severe danger. This reduction may be the result of a loss of blood through a break in the skin, a constriction of the blood vessels, or a loss of body fluids that rush to nourish some injured part of the body.

This last is the case with shock due to burns. Body fluids are dispatched to the burned tissue to supply nourishment to the cells. These fluids seep through the skin and are lost. If they are not quickly replaced through transfusions, the body's process can be so impaired by lack of blood supply that death soon follows. Shock is, therefore, the most important single consideration in the first moments after a victim incurs a severe burn.

Many physicians rely heavily upon extra doses of proper food elements in treating burns: a high protein intake is generally considered essential to the cure of burns, and as much as 400 grams of protein per day may be prescribed, and with it, 1 gram of ascorbic acid (vitamin C) daily, and large doses of the B vitamins.

The burn patient's nutritional state is of extreme im-

[84]

portance so that healing can come from within. The use of drugs often closes wounds superficially, then they show infection at a later time and must be treated by grafts and diet.

One of the nutrients hailed specifically for its effectiveness in treating burns is vitamin E (alpha tocopherol). Wilfred E. Shute, M.D., in his book "Vitamin E For Ailing and Healthy Hearts" (Pyramid), writes: "I have learned that vitamin E is of maximum use in treating burns, from the small domestic burn, due to contact with a heated iron or a stove burner or scalding steam and water, to the most severe third degree burns. Here the results are more important, because the scars that result from vitamin E treatment are unique and uniformly render unnecessary the usual costly, protracted skin grafting with resultant pain and agony to the patient."

Dr. Shute's experience in using vitamin E to treat severe burns involved a boy of six who suffered a second degree burn to the dorsum of the fingers of his left hand from a hot laundry iron. His father called, not to discuss his treatment, but to find out which of the local surgeons should be entrusted with the care and grafting of the burned hand, particularly important in this case because the child was left-handed. Instead, Dr. Shute treated the boy at home with 300 units of alpha tocopherol by mouth, since this was before there was such a preparation as vitamin E ointment.

The result was excellent. There was no infection and no deepening of the damaged tissue, i.e., only the tissue killed by the heat of the iron was lost. Healing was

[85]

rapid, and the resulting scar did not contract and was never tender. The boy regained completely normal function. He was not hospitalized and needed no skin grafting or other surgery, because there was no injury to the living tissue just below the necrotic tissue, and so no involvement of the tendons or tendon sheaths immediately below.

Another boy of six was badly scalded by a kettle of boiling water and he suffered multiple burns over his neck, torso, back and front, and left thigh. He was in the hospital for ten weeks. A skin grafting operation was performed but it was not successful, and the whole area became grossly infected. There were large raw areas, and frequent dressings were required. There was no evidence of healing except at the ends of the burn on the thigh; and here the scar seemd to be heaped up and contracted.

By this time alpha tocopherol ointment was available and, alternating with an antibiotic ointment, was used directly on the wound. The boy was also given 300 units of alpha tocopherol a day by mouth. The infection cleared up in the first four days. After ten days of treatment, only the vitamin E ointment was used, and there was complete healing in 13 weeks.

Dr. Shute planned to have any necessary skin grafting done sometime later. However, every time he saw the boy the skin had grown in still further. Ultimately Dr. Shute found that grafting need not be done.

Here again the unique characteristics of scars formed under alpha tocopherol therapy were evident. Whereas the scar formed on the thigh when the boy was

[86]

first seen was heaped up, the scar formed with alpha tocopherol was smooth and nontender. Moreover, there was no scar tissue contraction. The areas of healed scar were exactly the same size as the open wounds were when first seen.

In their search for new and better ways to handle burns, doctors have discovered special values in one of the basic compounds of the earth—salt. The *New York State Journal of Medicine* has stated that drinking a solution made of one level teaspoonful of common table salt and one-half teaspoonful of baking soda in a quart of water is as effective in emergency burn cases as is the administration of blood plasma. Several quarts of this saline solution must be consumed each day by the patient, in fact as many as he possibly can drink. Since burn victims always exhibit an unquenchable thirst the patient willingly drinks enough, especially if other beverages are refused him.

One consequence of severe injuries from burns is to force potassium out of damaged cells and sodium from the blood stream into them. The excess potassium then meanders through the body, slowing down heart action. At the same time, in order to replace the sodium lost to the cells, the blood stream taps its own reservoirs of salt water. This results in falling blood pressure, kidney slow-up and even fainting spells. Drinking literally gallons of saline solution (adults with severe burn have spontaneously swilled down more than 10 quarts in a twenty-four-hour period) enables the blood stream to replenish its stock of sodium, blood pressure goes up again and the kidneys speed up in pumping

[87]

the potassium out of the body. It is all simply a matter of keeping the vital sodium-potassium-water balance of the body normal.

Fortunately, for most of us, our experience with burns is limited to the painful but minor consequences of contact with hot pots, matches and radiators. First aid remedies for these vary from house to house and doctor to doctor. Most people put some kind of grease over the burn, some do nothing and "let the air get at it," in spite of instinct which tells us to plunge the burn into cold water to take the heat away. The *American Medical Association* recommends ice water as the best first aid measure for burns covering up to 20% of the body.

Soak the burned area immediately in a basin containing tap water, ice cubes and a disinfectant. For burns of the head, neck, chest, etc., where immersion is impractical, apply towels chilled in a bucket of ice water. The cold treatment is continued until it can be stopped without return of pain—usually within 30 minutes to 5 hours. Although the primary injurious effect of the burn has taken place, the usual inflammatory process secondary to the burn can be reduced in degree and at times reversed by ice-water therapy. The time factor between injury and treatment determines the result. This treatment should be initiated at once. This would be far more effective first aid treatment than applying butter or grease which will only have to be painfully removed by the attending physician.

It is the major burns, second or third degree burns over a third or more of the body, that pose some of medicine's most difficult problems. Severe scarring and a crippling shrinkage of muscle tendons almost inevitably result. The pain frequently cannot be relieved by any means. But nature has some answers that seem to have escaped the attention of most medical men.

On April 19, 1966, an Oregon farmer named Clarence Phillips suffered a severe electrical burn. A detonating wire he was working with came in contact with a high voltage line. 345,000 volts of electricity ran through his body. When he was found, more dead than alive, he had second and third degree burns over 70 per cent of his skin surface. The skin had been completely burned away exposing the bone over several inches of his skull and the tendons of his right foot were laid bare.

It was Phillips' good fortune that he was brought to Dr. J. Otto George, and M.D. of Clatskanie, Oregon. Dr. George's treatment had Phillips out of the hospital in three months—a remarkably short period of time for this type of burn—and in a few more weeks Phillips was completely recovered.

There was scarring on less than 10 per cent of the original 1,000 inches of skin area that had been burned. This scarring occurred in those areas (such as the abdomen below the diaphragm) which were in constant motion and consequently could not heal as well. There was no loss of movement in any respect.

What is Dr. George's miraculous treatment? It is a lotion combining oils that people—plain people—have known for ages could soothe and heal burns. Fundamentally it is castor oil and cod liver oil. And it seems to work better in the treatment of severe burns than any drug yet devised.

The treatment was first developed by Dr. George 35 years ago when he worked for four years as a government physician in Alaska. Then a young graduate of the University of Oregon School of Medicine, Dr. George found himself as discontent as most doctors with the existing and highly unsatisfactory treatments for burns.

The Indians and Eskimos of Alaska treated their own burns with cod liver oil, seemingly with greater success than doctors could achieve. Dr. George began experimenting with those oils that had a reputation for reducing the pain of burns and facilitating the healing process. Eventually he came up with his combination, FRST.

Dr. George has treated literally hundreds of burn patients and is well-known throughout the state for skill and success with his treatment. He does not shun drugs. Severe burns are invariably accompanied by shock and for this the doctor uses the same plasma, glucose and saline injections that any practitioner would use. He has no objection at all to the use of narcotics for immediate relief of pain. But to treat the burned area itself, it is his combination of natural oils that he relies upon.

Instead of the gauze that is commonly used, Dr. George makes his dressings of thicknesses of the cotton fiber that comes in pound rolls. These are saturated with FRST and will hold the oil for 24 hours far better than

[90]

gauze can. They don't stick to the crusts that are formed over burns as gauze dressings tend to do.

Once the dressings have been applied, the combination of oils begins soothing the pain of the burn immediately and any further pain-relieving drugs are usually unnecessary.

So far as the federal government is concerned, the George treatment is still in the experimental stage. The Food and Drug Administration has no control over the individual treatments administered by individual doctors, but so far as sale of the combination of oils goes, has authorized it only for use on first degree (minor) burns. Approval of its distribution for treatment of major burns must wait for the extensive reports on the experimental use of the treatment.

Doctors are now using it experimentally and Dr. George has made it available for any additional doctors who wish to try it, subject to record keeping and reporting requirements of the FDA. Any doctor wishing a supply of the remedy and instructions in its use can request them of Dr. George whose address is simply Clatskanie, Oregon.

The government and the medical profession rightfully proceed with extreme conservatism. But there is a large section of the state of Oregon including many practicing physicians in the region and hospitals as well, who are convinced, that by turning to the natural methods, Dr. George has come up with one of the best treatments for burns ever discovered.

Preventing burns is easier and less painful than treating them: It is sad to report that 70 per cent of all burns occur in or near the home and involve children under five years of age. The number one cause of these fires is clothing which becomes inflamed when it brushes burning trash, a fireplace or is ignited in that most fascinating and disastrous of all childhood games, playing with matches. Because they are fuller and frillier, girls' clothes more often figure in accidents of this type. It is up to the parents to see that their children learn to respect fire and to stay away from it. It is hard to think of any time in a child's life when there is a need for him to deal with fire: oil lamps and gas lights are no more; fireplaces, which are rare, should never be lighted by children and should be kept screened when burning. Most furnaces are now automatically fired and a child need not even be aware of their existence.

As for the ever-present fascination that matches seem to exert, the problem must be met before trouble starts. The child must be made to realize that matches are out of the domain of his playthings, that they are not to be touched by him. After you feel that this lesson has been carefully impressed upon the child, resolve to keep temptation out of his way. Remove all matches from places accessible to him, and make sure that they are not left by someone else in a place he might be able to reach.

It is difficult to exaggerate the dangers of hot liquids when children are around. A few basic precautions can prevent tragedy. First of all, keep children out of the kitchen when hot liquids are being handled; children can easily bump or trip you and the hot stuff might

[92]

spill down on them. If your stove is such that the handles to cookpots can protrude over the edge, always make certain that the handles are turned in, toward the back of the stove. A child's finger, tipping a pan in curiosity, can lead to a serious accident. Don't let children try their hand at cooking unless you can spare the time to supervise and give them your full attention. Stoves and children are a hazardous combination.

Chapter XI

Shingles

First you have the pain—often of great severity. If it's in your chest, you may come to the despairing conclusion that you're suffering a heart attack.

Or, if the pain throbs in the abdomen, you may be convinced that you have appendicitis. And a doctor might even agree with you! We are told by a medical man who ought to know that "not a few surgeons have been embarrassed by the appearance of the tell-tale rash the day after removal of a normal appendix."

The "tell-tale rash"—localized concentration of chicken-pox-like blebs or blisters appearing a few days after the pain commences—provides the doctor with a positive basis for diagnosis: the patient is suffering from shingles. The more formal medical term is herpes zoster—an infection of a major sensory nerve by the herpes zoster virus. The affected nerve (and accompanying rash) is most commonly on the chest or waist —hence the name zoster from the Greek word for girdle. However, the virus sometimes attacks nerves in the face, and serious complications can develop if the eye becomes involved.

The pain of the inflamed nerve (actually a form of neuralgia) can be excruciating—"exquisite pain" as some doctors describe it. Often it is accompanied by excessive sensibility of the skin, so that even the touch of clothing is unbearable. For some patients the pain is less severe, rather a dull nagging or burning sensation.

But one of the worst things about the pain of shingles is that it can linger on long after the active attack is over and the blisters have disappeared. Such long-lasting pain is not typical of the disease; but when it does happen, it seems to follow shingles in older people. Some 30 per cent of patients over 40 experience lingering pain, and among patients over 70, about 50 per cent have pain for a year or more. Young people usually recover from a shingles attack in a week or two, or a month at the most.

"It is fair to say that most standard text books come to the conclusion that there is as yet no specific treatment for herpes zoster which has been proved successful, and the best a doctor can do for his patient is to relieve pain with analgesic drugs, and possibly apply some surface treatment to minimize or prevent secondary infection of the skin lesions," writes Dr. J. A. C. Bamford and colleagues in an article on "The Natural History of Herpes Zoster" (*Medical Journal of Australia,* March 30, 1968).

"No specific therapy has been devised for herpes zoster," agrees Dr. Charles M. Wilhelmj, Jr., in *Postgraduate Medicine,* September 1969. "Treatment involves a number of supportive measures."

And the popular medical columnist, Dr. Joseph A. Molnar, states: "There is no specific cure for shingles,

[95]

just as there is no cure for a cold. You have to let the attack wear itself out."

Now, Dr. Molnar's comment should alert us to the possibility that—despite the medical profession's failure to date to come up with the "perfect pill" to counteract herpes zoster—there may very well be other non-traditional methods that will work. For the common cold, we now know from evidence assembled by Linus Pauling, doesn't *have* to "wear itself out," it can be stopped in its tracks by adequate doses of vitamin C.

Similarly, there is case history evidence (though no double-blind clinical tests) that vitamin C given in massive doses can limit the infection of shingles. Vitamin B_{12} has also been used with good results by a number of practitioners—even the standard physician's guide, the *Merck Manual,* cites reports that there is improvement in shingles following large doses of this B vitamin.

But, beyond these two vitamins that have been used specifically as treatments for shingles, the rest of the B complex (and some minerals as well) are of great importance in maintaining a healthy nervous system. It is reasonable to suggest that these nutrients could help to repel a viral attack on nerve cells. And it is equally reasonable to suppose that they would be beneficial in healing the damaged nerves that continue to cause pain after the active phase of the disease is over.

Of all viral diseases, it seems that shingles should be among the most responsive to nutrition therapy, which aims to build the body's own natural defenses against

[96]

infection and disease. We say this because of the very peculiar nature of the virus involved.

What makes this virus unusual is that it is identical with the virus (varicella) that causes chicken-pox. (Modern electron microscopic examination of viruses recovered from skin blisters of both diseases, plus blood serum tests of patients with both diseases, have provided convincing evidence of this fact.) It's called the varicella-zoster virus.

How one and the same virus can cause two absolutely distinct diseases, is explained by Dr. Bamford in the above-mentioned *Medical Journal of Australia:* "The currently accepted view is that chicken-pox is the response of the non-immune host to this virus, and shingles the response of the partially immune." In other words, when the virus first infects a person, usually in childhood, the result is chicken-pox; he is now immune to that disease but not to the virus's second line of attack.

You can catch shingles from contact with chicken-pox, but most cases of shingles occur without any such exposure. And herein lies the reason why a nutritional approach to combatting this disease holds particular promise.

Presumably the virus is present in everyone who has ever had chicken-pox. But most of us are able to keep that dormant virus dormant. Occasionally, some breakdown in normal body defenses permits the virus to "wake up" and inflict its second-round damage. This thesis is borne out by the fact that a large number of adverse conditions (which tend to break down na-

[97]

tural resistance) can initiate an attack of shingles: injury, debilitating disease, certain drugs (particularly the immunosuppressive medications), and a variety of poisons—for example, poisoning by carbon monoxide.

In other words, it's not the presence of the virus—which has been there all along—but the weakness or susceptibility of the host that is responsible for this disease. Theoretically, nutritional supplementation should rally the body's own defenses. Does this theory work in actual practice?

Let's look at vitamin C treatment first. The most dramatic results with this agent have been achieved by the North Carolina physician, Dr. Fred Klenner. In a paper published in *Southern Medicine and Surgery* (July 1949), Klenner wrote specifically about his experience in using vitamin C against the herpes zoster virus. There were eight shingles patients treated in the series he reported—all of whom were injected with 2 to 3 grams of ascorbic acid every 12 hours, plus 1 gram by mouth every two hours.

"Seven experienced cessation of pain within two hours of the first injection," he reported, "and remained so without the use of any other analgesic (pain-killing) medication. Seven of these cases showed drying of the vesicles (blisters) within 24 hours and were clear of lesions within 72 hours." The eighth case, a diabetic, took longer and required 14 injections (as compared to the average six injections given to the others), but she too was symptom-free within two weeks.

"One of the patients," Dr. Klenner wrote, "a man of 65, came to the office doubled up with abdominal pain and with a history of having taken opiates for the preceding 35 hours. He gave the impression of having an acute surgical condition. A massive array of vessicles extended from the dorsal nerve roots to the umbilicus, a hand's breadth wide. He was given 3000 mg (3 grams) of vitamin C intravenously and directed to return to the office in 4 to 5 hours. It was difficult to convince him that his abdominal pain was the result of his having 'shingles.' He returned in 4 hours completely free of pain. He was given an additional 2000 mg of vitamin C, and following the schedule given above he recovered completely in 3 days."

Now, this one physician's experience is certainly no hard-and-fast proof that vitamin C will always work so magically. Shingles hits with varying severity, and many patients do recover quickly without any medication at all. Nevertheless, it is very persuasive testimony that this vitamin can cut the infection short— and thereby not only relieve immediate discomfort but prevent scarring and fibrosis of the nerve which causes the lingering pain of post herpetic neuralgia.

The logic of vitamin C's usefulness against the herpes zoster virus lies in its general property as a detoxicant—an agent that reinforces the hundreds of defenses the body naturally possesses against poisons and infecting agents.

In dealing with shingles, it would be wise for the scientific world to test the efficacy of massive doses of vitamin C in large-scale clinical experiments, instead of relying on really dangerous drugs, such as steroids, used routinely with antibiotics by many physicians, and the anti-viral drug, cytosine arabinoside, which is now being used experimentally in severe cases of herpes zoster at Stanford University (*Medical World News,* May 21, 1971).

Vitamin B_{12} supplementation has also been found effective against shingles, as might be expected, since neurological damage is one manifestation of vitamin B_{12} deficiency. A number of physicians going back to Dr. K. E. Jolles writing in the *British Medical Journal* in 1955, have reported on speedy response to vitamin B_{12} injections. In one of the more recent reports, appearing in *The Indian Practitioner,* July 1967, Drs. A. K. Gupta and H. S. Mital, wrote that they observed "a dramatic response to vitamin B_{12} therapy as judged by relief of pain and the speed of disappearance of vesicles" in a group of 21 herpes zoster patients.

Improvement usually began, they say, on the 2nd or 3rd day of daily injections of 500 mcg of the vitamin. Follow-up study showed no development of post-herpetic neuralgia in any of the cases.

Again, though this therapy has not been proved in controlled tests, it seems to carry great promise. Certainly, if you should suddenly feel the pain of shingles and find the tell-tale rash breaking out, it would be wise to ask your doctor to try vitamin treatment at once—for the sooner therapy starts, the better the chance of complete recovery.

Of course, if you have had shingles in the past but are still suffering from the pain of post-herpetic neuralgia, there is no longer the possibility of "fighting the virus." For the virus has done its damage and is gone.

[100]

Pain-killing drugs are usually unsuccessful for this ailment, the medical text books tell us. In severe cases, where the pain is intolerable, surgery is sometimes used to cut the root of the nerve.

But perhaps the most important thing is to improve your nutrition, so that any damaged nerves are given the utmost support in healing. There are certain nutrients of particular value for the nerves, predominantly the B vitamins. We have already noted the importance of B_{12}. But every single element of the B complex is "particularly important to central nervous system activity," according to the noted vitamin specialist, Dr. David Coursin, speaking at a recent meeting at the Massachusetts Institute of Technology. Dr. Coursin also included vitamin C in this category.

Two minerals that should get your special attention are calcium and magnesium. As Dr. W. A. Krehl pointed out in *Nutrition Today* (September, 1967), "Magnesium deficiency unquestionably causes changes in nerve conduction, transmission at the myoneural junction and muscular contraction." And calcium, according to Drs. Ferris Pitts, Jr., and James McClure, Jr., writing in the *New England Journal of Medicine* (December 21, 1967), combines with lactate around the sensitive endings of the nerves, preventing the acid from irritating the nervous system. Calcium also is necessary for the transmission of nerve impulses.

So eat a diet rich in vitamin C, the B-complex and the minerals calcium, phosphorus and magnesium. Remember, that shingles virus is always present in your

[101]

body if you've ever had chicken-pox, and only your own good health and the health of your nerve cells keep this enemy at bay.

Chapter XII

Acne

Gail C. of Irvington, New Jersey, didn't go to her senior prom last year. She told her parents she just didn't feel like it, that it was a silly waste of time. They believed her. But the night of the prom, while her parents were visiting with neighbors, Gail locked herself in her bedroom and cried her heart out for hours. Gail has a vivacious personality, the kind of girl who is a lot of fun to be with. And a couple of years ago she was a pretty girl. But now her face is marred by pimples and blackheads.

Everybody understands that acne can be disastrous for a girl, but adults are less likely to appreciate the difficulty acne can cause for teenage boys. Dates are hard to get—sometimes impossible. Job interviews are usually a dead end. Posing for yearbook pictures can be traumatic.

Acne is so common among teenagers that they consider it as one of the unpleasant but necessary facts of life. Even Britain's medical journal, *The Lancet,* has referred to acne as "almost a normal accompaniment of puberty." It is usually considered a minor disease, at least physically. Psychologically, acne can be among the most crippling.

Desperate teenagers resort to any number of fad acne treatments; in fact, the number of quack remedies

[103]

for acne rivals those for the better publicized diseases, arthritis and cancer.

In recent years, x-ray has been used as a treatment —even though most experts are strongly opposed to radiation exposure except in life-or-death situations. Some doctors administer broad-spectrum antibiotics— tetracycline has been in use continually for several years—although there is no real evidence of their effectiveness. Now oral contraceptives are being given to female teenagers to help them fight acne.

Some years ago, Dr. Edmund D. Lowney of the University of Pennsylvania, tried minor surgery as an acne therapy. One of his colleagues reported success in treating acne with activated charcoal tablets. Another specialist blamed acne on extensive dreaming and lack of refreshing sleep. Still another dermatologist insisted that, ". . . in many cases successful therapy may well depend on treatment of the underlying unhappiness."

Since acne occurs most commonly at adolescence, it is generally accepted that the gland changes taking place at that time must have something to do with it. Sex hormones are developing; a child's body is becoming the body of an adult. There is abundant evidence that a diet lacking in certain vitamins and minerals can lead to acne. Unfortunately little effort is made among physicians and health agencies to *prevent* acne by educating parents and children to anticipate these needs.

Dermatologist generally treat acne externally. They prescribe lotions, or a combination of lotions with

X-rays or sunbaths. Sulfur, quartz lamps, lotio alba, tincture of green soap, hot or cold compresses—any of these might be a daily ritual for an acne sufferer, who usually goes right on developing more and more pimples.

Most doctors agree that the tried and true old-time remedies work as well as any. A recent bulletin from the Kansas State Department of Health reported that, according to one doctor, "Twenty-five per cent of acne can be managed successfully by washing the face four or five times a day . . ." But this cleansing should *not* be done with soap. The sebaceous glands are irritated by soap, and the irritation causes the glands to secrete still more sebum than normal. This excessive secretion is what creates the unsightly blotches and blackheads characteristic of acne.

The irritative qualities of soap, and the harsh effect it has on the skin have been demonstrated frequently in medical literature. Why presume that these objectionable qualities are suspended when soap is used on the face?

The best of the old-time acne therapies still seems the best today—vitamin A. And perhaps the most exciting therapy of all for acne is vitamin A in its acid form. This is not taken orally, but applied directly to the skin (topically).

For those new to vitamin A acid therapy, the early weeks of treatment may prove a disappointment. The acne seems to be aggravated. Scores of new comedones, or plugs in the pores, stud the skin surface and can be wiped away with the fingers. Slight pimples develop

[105]

into full-blown and open comedones. New pustules and papules suddenly appear. This condition continues for about six weeks. The explanation, according to researcher James E. Fulton, M. D., is that, "Under the influence of vitamin A acid, comedones, inert for weeks or months, suddenly 'blew-up.' As a rule, these inflammatory lesions were rather small, implying that the acid was exciting inflammatory explosions at an earlier stage than would occur naturally." Vitamin A's value against acne, said Fulton, lies in its action to control "hyperkeratosis of the sebaceous follicles."

Simply put, acne begins when the tiny channel or follicle leading from a sebaceous (oil) gland in the skin to the skin surface becomes plugged up. Ordinary dirt can plug it up, but far more frequently skin cells themselves are responsible.

The top layer of skin, epidermia, also called the *stratum corneum,* is hard and horny. Ordinarily these outer skin cells are continually being brushed away by clothing, bathing, etc. But during adolescence, for some reason, they tend to adhere to each other. Then, instead of being sloughed off, they lodge in the small follicles leading from the sebaceous glands.

Each hard little plug is known as a comedone. The plugged condition is called keratosis. When an individual has lots of comedones he is said to be suffering from hyperkeratosis of the sebaceous ducts or follicles.

The sebaceous glands ordinarily secrete a lubricant called sebum. Even when the follicle is plugged shut, the secretion continues. This causes swelling and irritation. A papule, or small pimple results. If the pimple contains pus, it is called a pustule. (sometimes a cyst forms.) In a typical acne case, that process is repeated hundreds of times on the face and neck. According to Fulton, vitamin A acid effectively reverses it.

Fulton and his superior, Albert M. Kligman, M. D., carried on their studies with 229 adolescent patients at the Acne Clinic, attached to the University of Pennsylvania. The patients were divided into four groups: 37 patients were given a traditional remedy, sulfur resorcinol, 49 received benzoyl peroxide, apparently the favorite acne treatment among most doctors; 40 more were control subjects. Vitamin A acid was used on the remaining 103 patients.

Every week the patients came to the clinic, and the number of comedones, papules, pustules and cysts were carefully counted. Between three and four months later, the degree of improvement was evaluated.

Results were impressive. Among the controls, there was a total improvement of 8.3 per cent—presumably, this is a natural rate of improvement without therapy. Of those on the sulfur-resorcinol, total improvement averaged 15.9 per cent. Those receiving bensoyl peroxide, the current medical favorite, showed 31.9 per cent improvement.

On vitamin A acid, improvement virtually doubled —to 61.9 per cent. And almost 40 per cent of these secured an excellent result.

But vitamin A acid is no cure-all for acne. Most patients are improved, but not all, and not everyone can tolerate the irritant effect. Furthermore, if the application of vitamin A is stopped, the acne will probably return, usually within three to six weeks. However, Dr. Jon D. Straumfjord, originator of the treatment, says that oral vitamin A supplements may keep acne away, once the condition is cleared up and the acid applications are discontinued.

Daily oral doses of vitamin A and diets high in that nutrient combined with soapless face-washing several times daily may spare youngsters now entering adolescence the misery of an acne condition.

Many years ago—at about the time vitamin A therapy was first discussed—vitamin D was receiving attention as an acne treatment. Unfortunately it is almost completely ignored today.

Back in 1940, Dr. Merlin Maynard of San Jose, California, reported on vitamin D and calcium for acne in the *Archives of Dermatology and Syphilis*. He studied 70 patients in one series and 60 in another, all treated with vitamin D; 75.6 per cent had satisfactory results in the first series and 83.4 per cent in the second series. In addition to receiving vitamin D, Dr. Maynard's patients followed a special diet, accenting lean meats, fresh fruits and green vegetables, with a minimum of carbohydrates; no sweets, chocolate, pastries, greasy or highly seasoned foods or soda fountain drinks.

Dr. Maynard concludes that, "The greatest benefit of using vitamin D in acne, in my opinion, has been the avoidance of roentgen therapy (X-ray) which too often becomes the master rather than the servant of the physician. And certainly my satisfaction with vitamin D treatment has been great. The other vitamins

[108]

have an irrefutable place, but their use is by no means as general as vitamin D."

In spite of this optimistic report, little meaningful research on vitamin D and acne has appeared since.

What about other vitamins in acne therapy? Wallace Marshal, M. D., of Mobile, Alabama, treated a number of cases with liver extract and found moderate or marked improvement in 68 per cent of the patients. A different liver preparation used in a later study brought moderate or marked improvement to 89 per cent of the acne sufferers. There was also a beneficial action on the menstrual periods of women and girls taking the treatment.

Dr. Marshall experimented with liver extract for healing acne scars in seven patients. Over a period of seven months to two years, scars became less noticeable, skin became softer and thinner; scars which had been hard ridges softened considerably.

In addition to vitamins A and D liver also contains large amounts of the B complex, calcium, phosphorus, iron and copper.

Vitamin C's role in *controlling* acne was demonstrated by Dr. George E. Morris of Boston. He found that 43 of 53 acne patients showed improvement after 4 months of receiving two 8-ounce glasses of citrus juice and 3 grams of ascorbic acid each day.

Dr. Samuel M. Bluefarb of Northwestern University has found that a combination of 1 gram of vitamin C, orange juice—plus 100,000 units of vitamin A administered daily—benefits adolescent acne.

Paul Kline, M.D., treated 25 patients with multivitamin injections over a period of eight months. Twenty-four of the patients responded with satisfactory improvement. There was very little tendency of the acne to return after the injections were stopped. The younger the patients, the better their response.

Louis Tulipan, M.D., of New York, believes that vitamin B deficiency is the main cause of acne rosacea, a form of the disease prevalent among adults of 25 to 45 years old. The skin thickens and becomes bright, purplish-red over the nose and on the cheeks and chin. Vitamin B shortages sometimes occur even in persons who eat a perfectly balanced diet, because the digestive tract fails to assimilate certain kinds of food. Diet supplements can work wonders in such cases.

After observing 96 patients over a period of eight years, Dr. Tulipan is convinced that vitamin B deficiency is the primary cause of acne rosacea. He credits his success in treating this ailment to using brewer's yeast which contains all the B complex of vitamins, rather than using just one or the other of the B vitamins alone.

These encouraging results with vitamin therapy are reported in medical journals, but rarely come to the attention of the public. Instead, the public is exposed to material such as this, taken from the November 1961 issue of *Today's Health* (an organ of the American Medical Association). In an article, ironically titled "All About Acne," Dr. Bruce Bairstow answers teenagers' questions:

QUESTION: Why does it (acne) affect some but not others?

ANSWER: This is determined, probably, more by heredity than anything else. If your parents were fairly clear of acne, your chances are probably greater of staying clear.

QUESTION: How can we prevent acne?

ANSWER: Strictly speaking, it can't be prevented. However, it can be treated. At the first sign of acne, active treatment can be instituted to keep it suppressed until one outgrows it.

QUESTION: Does a controlled diet help?

ANSWER: Acne is not caused by faulty diets, although certain foods will make it worse. . . .

In the question and answer session, there was not one word about vitamin deficiency, nothing about improving the diet (except the well-worn vague advice about avoiding carbohydrates, fats, and sweets), and nothing about vitamin therapy.

Dr. L. Edward Gaul suggested in *The Journal of the Indiana State Medical Association* (January, 1966) that excessive use of salt may be related to acne. Adolescents on low salt diets have shown improvement within two weeks, and in two months, the acne bumps disappear entirely, according to Gaul. His article points out that adolescents get excessive salt with such popular snacks as french fries, popcorn and potato chips. It is worth noting that all of these snacks are

[111]

also heavy on residual hydrogenated fats. One girl of 17, pleased with her cleared complexion, told the doctor, "My snacking days are over."

Few adolescents are willing to forego snacking entirely. But snacking habits can be improved to satisfy ever-active appetites and provide nutrition at the same time, by including fresh or dried fruits, nuts and raw vegetables.

Chapter XIII

Athlete's Foot

"My war with athlete's foot began when I was in Washington, D.C., about 1920-21," wrote J. I. Rodale in the December, 1964, issue of *Prevention* magazine. "My feet itched badly. I was told that it was due to walking bare-foot in gymnasium shower rooms.

"For 15 years I visited doctors and clinics, and tried many patent salves and ointments but the itch continued on. After a while I gave up hope and resigned myself to my regular before bed scratch. Around about 1937 I noticed a new type of shoe being sold, perforated with little holes in the uppers, and bought a pair. Upon leaving the store I noticed immediately the invigorating feel of the wind between my toes. And miracle upon miracle, in 2 or 3 days the itching disappeared, and the raw condition of the skin between my toes healed up nicely. But I kind of missed the nightly scratch."

Quite by accident, Mr. Rodale had stumbled across one of the most effective means of treating athlete's foot—plain, ordinary air. Doctors have known for some years now that athlete's foot is not highly contagious as formerly believed. According to the Lehigh County (Pa.) Medical Society:

"Athlete's foot usually occurs on the feet when they remain sweaty for a long time. The skin is softened

[113]

and the viruses which are very common and usually found on the feet get hold under the skin. Because the feet of athletes and sportsmen often are perspired, the disease has become known as athlete's foot and has been supposed to be spread in lockers and barracks. Actually, it is wool and nylon socks which do not absorb perspiration that encourage the disease together with heavy leather or rubber shoes.

"During World War II athlete's foot was the second most common skin disease and caused 10 per cent of the hospital cases. Heavy shoes, wet for days, accounted for much of this. The army issues only cotton socks unless in very cold climates in order to avoid this problem.

"A survey in a university showed that 80 per cent of the men had athlete's foot, but only 15 per cent of the women. It was considered due to the fact that the women wore light shoes and light stockings.

"All in all, the important thing is to keep the skin of the feet in good condition. In the summer it is a good idea to go barefooted occasionally, not for the sake of the sun, but to build up more resistance in the skin due to exposure to the fresh air."

Mr. Rodale, writing on athlete's foot again in March, 1965, added another interesting observation: "In my own experience I found that the emotions had something to do with itching of the toes. Why did it always come at night when I took my shoes off, and never in the daytime? Correction! I recall it happening in the daytime once when I delivered a speech on organic gardening at Haddon Heights, N.J., when I had been asked a lot of difficult questions! Perhaps it is the excessive sweating that is induced by anxiety that does it."

Some years ago, Drs. Stokes and Pillsbury, dermatologists at the University of Pennsylvania Medical School, said, "The larger our experience, the more careful our search, the more we are inclined to believe that in the urticarias (hives) . . . in (certain types of) eczemas . . . even in dermatoses which, like athlete's foot, seem far removed from psychologic considerations, the tension, the conflict and anxiety, have their place as casual influences to be sought out and rectified side by side with, and sometimes even before, the correction of the more apparent physical dysfunctions."

Dr. William S. Becker, of the University of Chicago, said in a lecture that recent medical research indicates that the disease may be due to nervous exhaustion and inability to relax properly.

What seems likely is that, whether from sweat, nervous perspiration or any number of causes, moisture accumulates on the feet. If this moisture is not absorbed into socks or evaporated into the air, fungi will begin to grow and actually thrive in the warm, dark moisture and feast on the skin—especially between the toes.

In the past, doctors would advise regular washing of the feet—usually with soap. The more the patients washed, though, the more severe the ailment became. To start with, the soap irritated the already sensitive

[115]

skin, making it even easier for the fungus to destroy the skin tissue. But even if soap was not used, the people who washed their feet would fail to dry them properly. The irritation was painfully sensitive, so they would simply dry the areas *surrounding* the sore spot. The result was that more moisture was available for the fungus to thrive on. And thrive they did.

This matter of not drying the feet carefully after a bath is probably the leading cause of athlete's feet. The treatment is as simple as the cause: Dry the feet very carefully after bathing—particularly between the toes. Then, keep them dry. Wear only cotton socks. They absorb moisture. The stretch socks made of nylon and other synthetic fibers, are particularly unacceptable. Change socks frequently, if necessary, but keep the feet dry at all costs.

And finally, let your feet and the spaces between your toes be exposed to the air as often as possible. You needn't wear shoes and socks in your home, so, if you have athlete's foot, go barefoot.

Following this advice, you might get rid of athlete's foot in a week or less; perhaps, with care, you can avoid getting it ever again.

Chapter XIV

Eczema

To a great extent, eczema is a disease of infants and children. It is a skin disease identified by dry-appearing patches of skin, crusted and scaly with cracks or breaks that sometimes "weep." The rash produces a severe itching and burning in the affected area.

Medical Times carried an article some years ago, describing the experience of investigator B. M. Kesten, who studied 2,000 cases of eczema and found that about two-thirds of this group were less than 6 years old and the largest concentration of patients was between 9 and 24 months of age.

The September 1959 issue of the *Journal of The American Dietetic Association* says that certain kinds of eczema may improve with pyridoxine (vitamin B₆) treatment, even after other treatments have failed. Dr. W. A. Krehl of Yale University, author of the article states that good results have been achieved when 24 to 50 mgs. of pyridoxine are given intravenously or subcutaneously, but that "many of these cases of seborrheic dermatitis responded well to the local application of pyridoxine."

Bicknell and Prescott, in their book *Vitamins in Medicine,* tell of many cases where ingesting unsaturated fatty acids greatly improved eczema. What are unsaturated fats? They are the ones that stay liquid at

[117]

room temperature. The oil you use in salad dressings is unsaturated. So are the liquid cooking oils (soybean oil, wheatgerm oil, sunflower seed oil, corn oil, etc.).

Since the earliest investigations, in 1933, researchers have known that unsaturated fats can be used to treat eczema. Lee Foundation Report (February, 1942) reported that 87 chronic eczema patients, who were seen over a four and a half year period, responded to treatment with corn oils, though standard treatments used for years had failed. *The American Journal of Diseases of Children* (January, 1947) issued a similar report on 171 children suffering from eczema and treated with unsaturated fatty acids. About half of these (none of whom has shown any response to other treatments) improved markedly.

Another approach to treating eczema, now used in vogue in Russia, is vitamin A from pumpkins. In *Abstracta Dermatologica* (September-October, 1965) Russian scientists reported that patients were given 20 to 40 drops of carotene (the provitamin that occurs naturally in yellow vegetables and is converted into vitamin A by the body) from stored pumpkins. This was taken twice daily by mouth, and an ointment made of the carotene was rubbed on the affected part of the skin. According to the abstract, "Apparent cures or considerable improvements were observed in 16 of 19 patients with eczema (including infant eczema), in 24 of 33 patients with microbial eczema . . . and in 6 of 7 patients with serious manifestations of hyperkeratosis (scaliness) of the skin."

[118]

If you are depending on your meals alone for vitamin A, remember that this vitamin usually occurs in foods as carotene, which must be made into vitamin A by the body. If, through some disorder, your system cannot make the conversion and you are not taking food supplements that contain vitamin A itself such as fish liver oils you might suffer from a deficiency. Diabetics, for example, are believed to be unable to transform carotene into vitamin A.

R. Patiala, M.D., of the University of Helsinki, Finland, conducted studies with vitamin B_2 and reported these findings in 1966: "For about three years I have undertaken partly in the cutaneous disease section of the clinic of the University of Helsinki, partly on the outside, the use of vitamin B_2 preparations in the treatment of infantile eczema and diathetic Besnier's prurigo (chronic itching skin inflammations).

"The patients studied represented five cases of severe infantile eczema, and 21 cases of Besnier's prurigo of which three were associated with attacks of asthma. The ages of the patients ranged between 6 and 12 months for the infantile eczema, between 3 and 32 years for prurigo.

"Of the subjects overtaken with prurigo, 17 were of the female sex and 4 of the masculine sex. One notes in the previous hereditary history of the majority of the patients some eczema, some asthma and occasionally both . . .

"The eczematous patients presented head and especially facial eruption, associated in some with an erup-

[119]

tion of the bend of the arms, of the elbows and of the back. The condition of the patients overtaken with Besnier's prurigo varied considerably in intensity according to the case, but all offered typical lesions at the bend of the arm and at the back of the knee and often at the lateral part of the neck. The hermatologic (blood) examination showed an eosinophil (white corpuscle count) varying from 4 to 10 per cent."

According to Dr. Patiala, treatment of these patients with vitamin B_2 offered excellent results. He outlined the evolution of the disease in one of the subjects:

Mrs. C., age 26, is the wife of a bank employee, and had been suffering since the age of six months with a disease considered at first to be infantile eczema and then recognized as diathetic prurigo. She has undergone all kinds of internal and external medications. Her condition was aggravated by a pregnancy. One noted neither asthma nor eczema in her heredity. The patient showed large oozing patches of the face, the bend of the elbow, the neck and the popliteal (rear knee) space; she manifested a condition of accentuated nervousness and was not able to tolerate a stay at the hospital.

The treatment prescribed consists of 25 ampules of 2 c.c. of riboflavin (vitamin B_2) administered intravenously at the rate of two ampules per day. Seven days after the end of the treatment the patient was much improved and the skin was dry and thin. A second series of riboflavin injections was prescribed 15 days after the end of the first, and at the same time

[120]

a local application of the vitamin in a watery paste. A month after this second series the patient declared that she had never been in such good condition in her life; the skin had again become thin and supple with only a light thickening perceptible on the bend of the elbows and popliteal space.

A pregnancy, occurring six months later, did not noticeably modify her health and inquiry made four years later revealed that the condition was maintained well with several passing relapses, which were cured in several weeks with topical applications of B_2

In all cases of infantile eczema, Dr. Patiala has administered vitamin B_2 by intramuscular route ($\frac{1}{2}$ to 1 ampule every two days according to age); the series was composed of five ampules. By contrast Besnier's prurigos were treated by intravenous route and as much as possible daily, at the rate of two ampules of riboflavin, or one ampule of lactoflavine. If necessary, a second identical series has been administered a month after the end of the preceding one and in some cases even a third after a delay of 2 to 3 months.

The tolerance has always been perfect; no patient has found discomfort even after the dose (exceptionally administered) of four ampules at one time. During the first five injections no local care was used. Then some creams or soothing pomades were applied. It is, furthermore, probable that a smaller dose of vitamin B_2, for example a half ampule two times per week, would have been sufficient.

The therapeutic action of riboflavin and of lactoflavine being identical, there is no place to separate the results that they give. Their rapid efficiency in the case of infantile eczema was evident; as early as the fourth day after the first injection the skin was dry, still a little scaly, but the improvement was still better characterized by the disappearance of itching; the infants, previously restless and agitated, ceased to scratch, remained quiet and slept again. When the treatment was undertaken at the acute phase, the cure occurred without relapse after a single series and with two children, without any additional local care.

In chronic eczemas of the type of Besnier's prurigo the improvement was manifested by the improvement in appearance of the outbursts of acute itching.

The action of vitamin B_2 on the nervous condition merits particular mention. Disappearance of restlessness and the return of sleep were particularly noted in the children of 7 to 9 years of age. This and a good appetite were considered the essential ingredients for improving the general condition. The cure obtained by the riboflavin or the lactoflavine has, however, been lasting only in two cases; in the other cases relapses occurred, but they were generally weaker than the initial attacks. In the three intricate cases of asthma with eczema, the asthma yielded first and improvement of the cutaneous symptoms followed.

Although lasting results have not always been obtained in infantile eczema and diathetic prurigo treated with riboflavin or lactoflavine, it is thus permissible to say that this medication represents a very important contribution in the treatment of these rebellious dis-

[122]

eases and that it aids the patients to recover from the extreme discomfort of attacks of acute itching.

Soy products seem to have some value in treating eczema. The January 10, 1957, issue of *Medical Science* carried Dr. Sidney Kane's observations on 102 infants, aged 1 week to 9 months, whose symptoms of asthma, eczema, nasal discharge, and irritability were traced to a sensitivity to cow's milk. After soy milk was substituted, 75 of the 76 infants with eczema improved greatly.

Always eat soybeans cooked, as raw soybeans contain a factor that inhibits trypsin, an important enzyme needed for protein utilization. Raw soybeans also interfere with growth by tying up such minerals as calcium and phosphorus in the body.

There are a number of ways to serve soybeans so that you do obtain optimum nutrition. You can steam them, bake them in the style of baked beans, mix them with corn or tomato sauce, or even roast the kernels, as you would roast peanuts. Soy milk makes a refreshing drink for everyone, and it is high in lecithin.

Chapter XV

Ichthyosis and Psoriasis

Ichthyosis is an especially unpleasant type of skin disease, characterized by widespread dry patches on the skin that turn dark and scaly. The skin, where it is affected, resembles fish skin in appearance, which is how the disease got its name: *ichthus* is Greek for *fish*.

American medicine has paid little attention to ichthyosis, although thousands suffer from it. It is nothing like a fatal disease. Its effects seem to be chiefly psychological, due to distress caused by the exceptionally ugly appearance it gives to the affected skin areas. Ichthyosis is in that class of diseases that seem to have been put in the world for the special benefit of dermatologists whose patients, legendarily, are never cured of their ailments and never die from them. The long held belief that ichthyosis is a hereditary and incurable disease is generally accepted among our physicians.

In Egypt, however, where ichthyosis is widespread and where the extreme dryness of the climate makes it far more uncomfortable, there is more pressure on doctors to produce a cure. After much experimentation, that is just what they have done.

In the *Egyptian Pharmaceutical Bulletin* (44, 4, April, 1962) Dr. M. R. Zawahry of Ain Shams University stated that "niacin is probably the most valuable therapeutic agent in ichthyosis. . . . Cases have been cleared entirely after a period of treatment with this vitamin. Such cases always recur when the treatment is discontinued. . ."

When a doctor is able to cure any disease by administering a nutrient and the disease recurs when the nutrient is discontinued it is reasonable to conclude that the disease is actually caused by a deficiency of the particular nutrient. The question then arises, is the deficiency due to insufficient amounts in the diet, or is it due to a physiological defect that makes it impossible to utilize the nutrient?

To answer this question, Dr. Zawahry checked the urine of a number of ichthyotic patients of various ages from 3 to 24, for N-methyl nicotinamide, the final stage of vitamin B_3 (niacin) in the body. He reasoned that if the vitamin, when eaten or administered, were eventually excreted in this form, then it must have gone through all the chemical transformations within the body that are necessary to proper metabolism of that vitamin.

Dr. Zawahry found, that while the original vitamin B_3 levels of the ichthyotic patients were low, administration of large doses resulted in perfectly normal serum levels and excretion that corresponded to expected levels of normalcy. So it was scientifically demonstrated that ichthyosis is probably due to a deficiency of niacin, and is not a hereditary fault in the metabolism.

Because it is similar to ichthyosis, psoriasis is looked upon as a cousin of that disease. Every day psoriasis

[125]

claims new sufferers—men and women throughout the country who look in the mirror and discover little red patches that weren't there before on their elbows and knees. The patches are covered by white or yellowish scales, which, if scratched, become silvery and flake off like dandruff. (Psoriasis of the scalp is often mistaken for dandruff.) Sometimes the red patches itch, sometimes not. But they are unsightly, and their name has become synonymous with embarrassment.

If you spot these symptoms in yourself and consult your doctor, you might be disappointed by his treatment. The medical profession acknowledges no definite cause for this unsightly disease, and no sure cure.

"Psoriasis is an antidote for the dermatologist's ego," P. Bechet, an eminent dermatologist and medical historian, once remarked. The pesky scaling disease drives its victims to try everything in the dermatologist's medicine bag—tar, mercury Chrysarobin, phenol—and some of these do bring a measure of relief. Then—boom! The eruptions are back in full bloom, bigger than ever, redder, itchier and more repulsive. Next the dermatologist might resort to X-ray therapy, which carries the risk of dangerous side effects.

While some doctors still use the coal tar or mercury ointments, it is the steroids, ACTH and cortisone, and their derivatives, that are most frequently prescribed today. These sometimes lead to problems worse than the original ailment. But some victims of psoriasis are so miserable that they willingly take the calculated risk inherent in the steroids. Unfortunately, any positive result is generally temporary. Steroids often lead to

[126]

severe recurrences and bad reactions. Cortisone causes urinary losses of calcium and phosphorus, resulting in demineralization of the bones which can become so porous that an exertion no stronger than a sneeze might break a rib. An added problem with steroid therapy is severe depression; it invites ulcers and adrenal exhaustion with a subsequent drain on recuperative powers. It also weakens the body's defenses so that dormant, forgotten infections can take hold once more.

A doctor may recommend some combination of salves, ointments and compresses to give short-term relief. Hopefully, however, he will also investigate the patient's diet.

Research indicates that psoriasis is, at least partially, a disease involving defective metabolism and a faulty diet. Of those experimenters who have treated the disease with any measure of success, many have concerned themselves chiefly with the elements of diet involved in fat metabolism.

Twenty years ago, Doctors Paul Gross and Beatrice M. Kesten, from the Department of Dermatology at the Columbia-Presbyterian Medical Center, reported success in treating psoriasis with soybean lecithin. (Lecithin supplements are almost always derived from the soybean plant.)

The doctors eliminated eggs, fat meats, poultry, fish, cheese and excessive amounts of butter and cream from their patients' diets in order to run the experiment on a strict low-fat regimen. The lecithin was distributed to the 235 subjects, along with vitamins A and D and the B vitamins thiamin, pyridoxine, riboflavin and pantothenic acid. Because of the restricted diet, the doctors considered it important to administer vitamin supplements, but felt certain the lecithin was responsible for the therapeutic results in this case. Out of the total figure the researchers considered that 155 were adequately treated. The rest either did not cooperate or abandoned the diet before any conclusions could be drawn.

Only 37 patients experienced no improvement. Twenty-three of the patients remained disease-free after one year of therapy and three years of observation. Of those remaining, 29 experienced satisfactory control of their psoriasis, and 66 subjects showed some improvement, but required therapeutic ointments in addition to the lecithin in order to bolster their progress.

Doctors Gross and Kesten concluded that "this form of therapy is capable of correcting some of the metabolic defects but not the actual cause of the disease." They recommend a low-fat diet, plus a lipotropic, or fat-emulsifying substance such as lecithin to control psoriasis, for the same reason that "proper diet and supportive treatment alone can control many cases of diabetes."

Faulty diet and defective metabolism may lead to psoriasis. But the relationship doesn't stop there. The skin disease may drain your body of essential nutrients and create a further deficiency in your body.

In 1965, Daphne Roe, M.D., a dermatologist and nutritionist at Cornell University, told the annual meeting of the New York State Medical Society that psoriasis may be more serious than is usually assumed. She warned that the constant loss of skin tissue can cause enormous losses of vitamin and mineral nutrients. Even people who eat a normally good diet, she said, might develop nutritional deficiencies in the wake of psoriasis.

At the same time Dr. Roe proposed dietary means to control this supposedly incurable disease. Studies at the Clinical Nutritional Unit of Cornell University suggest that psoriasis comes about because of a metabolic defect, probably in enzyme production, that renders the body unable to handle the amino acid taurine normally. Taurine is not one of the essential amino acids. It is formed within our own bodies. But apparently our bodies rarely, if ever, manufacture any excess taurine. Whenever there is too much of this amino acid in the system, it's from the foods we eat. If we lack the metabolic ability to take care of excess amounts of taurine properly psoriasis can result. In a convincing demonstration of this, the people at Cornell successfully rid a group of patients of psoriasis and the patients stayed well up to two years by sticking to a diet that was deliberately low in taurine.

Controlling taurine intake is difficult. Practically all proteins, from porterhouse steak to herring, contain substantial amounts of this amino acid. As Dr. Roe pointed out, protein is an absolutely essential food; you cannot dispense with it just to eliminate the taurine it contains.

The Cornell experimenters found that taurine is ex-

[129]

tremely susceptible to leaching in boiling water. By insisting that their patients boil all meats for at least five minutes, and throw away the cooking water before boiling, roasting or whatever else they intended to do with the food, they managed to eliminate most of the taurine contained in these meats.

This cooking method would hardly be recommended to anybody else. In terms of flavor and texture, boiling is usually the worst thing you can do to a piece of meat. Nutritionally speaking, it is absolutely sinful. Boiling removes most of the water soluble vitamins, which means the entire B complex and whatever vitamin C there may be in the food. It also leaches out important minerals.

In discussing the problem of finding a protein food with low taurine content, Dr. Roe said that such foods were being developed, and noted that soybean products "seem promising."

The use of B vitamins in treating psoriasis can't be ignored. *The Journal of Investigative Dermatology* reports that riboflavin (vitamin B_2) taken both orally and by injection, seems to help in some psoriasis cases. Dr. Merlin Maynard, who conducted the research, reported that this treatment healed lesions in 25 per cent of patients, and improved most of the rest. In some cases the beneficial results lasted for two years after the treatment was discontinued.

Dr. John F. Madden, an M.D. in St. Paul, Minnesota, has achieved good results in treating psoriasis with vitamin B_1 (thiamin), an ointment and a low-fat diet. Reporting in the *Journal of the American Medical*

[130]

Association, he said that, after experimenting with various treatments, vitamin B_1 was most beneficial, bringing definite improvement to one-third of the patients who tried it.

In addition to thiamin and riboflavin, some physicians report good results with vitamin B_{12}, when continued for as long as 30 days.

So far, we have found no mention in the medical literature of any experiments which used the entire B complex, in natural form, for the treatment of psoriasis. However, if thiamin helps one patient, riboflavin helps another, and B_{12} helps a third, we can infer that supplements such as desiccated liver and brewer's yeast —rich in the entire B complex—ought to help a large proportion of psoriasis sufferers.

Another "promising" treatment for psoriasis is vitamin A acid, the face-saver of the acne patient. In a double-blind controlled study, Phillip Frost, M.D., and Gerald D. Weinstein, M.D., of the Department of Dermatology, University of Miami School of Medicine, found that vitamin A, in its acid form, did indeed bring remarkable relief from the itching and unsightliness of psoriasis and ichthyosis in 24 out of 26 patients. These effects were noticeable after only one week of treatment. (*Journal of the American Medical Association,* March 10, 1969).

Before they undertook a clinical study of vitamin A acid, Dr. Frost and Dr. Weinstein first compared the effects of several commonly available forms of topically administered vitamin A (vitamin A acid, vitamin A aldehyde, vitamin A alcohol, and vitamin A acetate)

[131]

on three patients who had extensive psoriasis and three patients with ichthyosis. After one week, the area which had vitamin A acid applied to it showed markedly decreased scaling among the patients with the dry, rough, scaling skin of ichthyosis and much less redness among those patients with psoriasis. No changes were discernible where the other forms of vitamin A had been applied.

Intrigued by the superior healing properties demonstrated by this simple patch test, Frost and Weinstein then began a more extensive evaluation of vitamin A acid.

They chose patients with those skin conditions most resistant to all kinds of treatment—10 with epidermolytic hyperkeratosis, in which the skin becomes hard and loose; 24 with some form of ichthyosis and 26 with extensive psoriasis. Vitamin A acid scored major points in almost every patient, especially those with disorders which do not usually respond to the dermatologist's efforts. The improvement was dramatic in patients with psoriasis.

Frost and Weinstein point out that, to be effective, the vitamin A acid solution should be either a .2% or .3% concentration. When German investigator von Beer used a .1% vitamin A acid preparation on 20 patients, there was no noticeable improvement. The Florida investigators believe their more favorable response is due to the use of the higher concentrations. It is interesting to note that the improvement resulting from vitamin A acid usually lasted 10 to 14 days after discontinuing therapy.

[132]

It would be ideal if you could go to your drugstore for vitamin A acid. But, unfortunately, you won't find it there. You can't even get it from your doctor or dermatologist. As this is being written, vitamin A acid is going through FDA test requirements for safety and efficiency as an NDA (new drug applicant). And, unless the FDA's lengthy procedures and practices in handling new drug applications are considerably revised and improved, there is little likelihood that vitamin A acid will be available for victims of psoriasis for some time.

However, there is much that the patient with psoriasis can do to improve his health status while he is waiting for the vitamin A acid. Halibut liver oil is an excellent source of both vitamin A and its working partner, vitamin D, which might also have an ameliorative effect on psoriasis. D is the sunshine vitamin and it has been observed that psoriasis improves in the summer because of day to day exposure to the sun. It almost never appears on the face and hands, which are exposed to the sun more than the rest of the body.

Physicians have given 200,000 vitamin A units daily for six months, according to J. M. Lewis et al, writing in the *Journal of Pediatrics,* (31, 496, 1947) without observing any signs of toxicity. However, it is not considered advisable to take more than 50,000 units of vitamin A daily, unless you are being supervised by a physician.

Years ago it was determined that what sometimes seems to be a deficiency of vitamin A, may be a deficiency of vitamin E. Unless vitamin E is amply sup-

[133]

plied, the vitamin A obtained from both foods and supplements, the vitamin A already in the blood, and that which is stored in the liver and other body tissues, is quickly destroyed by oxygen. (*Biochemical Journal* 34, 1321, 1940).

To summarize, then, those bothered by psoriasis really should be conscious of every mouthful of food they eat. They should avoid meat and dairy fats. The only acceptable fats are unsaturated fats, such as those in eggs, salad oils and other vegetable sources such as sunflower seeds, avocados and raw nuts. Not only are they valuable for psoriasis, but they also help melt fat deposits and keep cholesterol emulsified, circulating and supplying energy instead of menacing health.

Patients should avoid hydrogenated shortenings, the thick white ones many people use for frying and baking. Margarine is also hydrogenated. Psoriasis sufferers will do well to shun the hidden fats which they are bound to encounter if they buy any packaged foods at all or if they eat in restaurants. Crackers are crisp because of the hydrogenated shortening they contain.

Food supplements can supply vitamins A and D (plentiful in fish liver oils), and the B vitamins (wheat germ, brewer's yeast or desiccated liver are the best sources), lecithin and/or the unsaturated fatty acids available in flakes or in capsules. These lecithin supplements, derived chiefly from soybeans, should be a staple in the diet of every psoriasis sufferer.

Chapter XVI

Vitiligo

Vitiligo is a painless skin disease which is character-ized by the disappearance of natural color, or pigment, from patches on the skin. Even the fairest skins have some color, and when it goes, these patches of abso-lute white are very definitely visible and can be most embarrassing. In a darker skin the problem is empha-sized.

Medical literature provides detailed descripitions of vitiligo; but there is little direction on what to do about it. Some years ago, Benjamin Sieve, M.D., former in-structor in medicine at Tufts Medical School, gave a comprehensive history of the treatments in use back in the 1930's and 1940's, and the then-current thinking on the subject. Very little seems to have been accom-plished in the treatment of vitiligo since then. The medical journals nowadays hardly even mention the problem.

Among the treatments described by Sieve is one used by H. W. Francis, M.D. He thought the disease was due to the absence of free hydrochloric acid in the stomach, since he had vitiligo and found the acid ab-sent in himself. He took 15 cc. doses of hydrochloric acid at each meal for 2 years and noted that the vitiligo areas completely disappeared. He used the same therapy on three other patients and reported similar results. Dr. Sieve suggested that the effect of the hydrochloric acid might have been to aid in processing and absorption of necessary nutrients.

The theory of nutrition as a factor in preserving skin pigment turned up in the *Archives of Dermatology and Syphilology* (March, 1937) where researchers told of using vitamin C to restore skin color. The following year a German medical journal carried an article also recommending vitamin C as a treatment for vitiligo.

Para-amino-benzoic acid (PABA), a B vitamin, has been mentioned repeatedly in connection with the treatment of vitiligo. M. J. Costello, in the *Archives of Dermatology and Syphililogy* (February, 1943) told of his success in treating vitiligo of the eyelids in a 2-year-old child with 100 mg. of PABA daily. Dr. Sieve was impressed with the potential of PABA, and set up an experiment to observe its effect on 48 cases of vitiligo.

The group consisted of 25 females and 23 males, ranging in age from 10 to 70 years. The vitiligo condition had persisted for from 2 to 28 years. Most of the patients showed evidence of a chronically poor diet and a history of gland imbalance. Fatigue, irritability and emotional instability were common among them, as were constipation, weight gain, arthritis and various types of headaches. Physical examinations presented classic findings consistent with an underactive thyroid condition in many of the subjects. Along with these came a preponderance of brittle nails, coarse and thick-

[136]

ened skin and varying degrees of hypertension (high blood pressure).

An accurate history of each patient was obtained, including blood counts, urine tests, blood sugar, basal metabolism, etc. The gland balance was established through the use of hormones. Then all patients were given a patent combination of B complex vitamins— more than the recommended daily dosage. In addition, PABA was administered in the form of 100 mg. tablets three or four times daily. This treatment continued for a period of ten months. The rate of improvement in the skin of those using oral PABA was slow. Some patients followed the described regimen for 18 weeks with no results.

Dr. Sieve instituted injections of the vitamin, coupled with monoethanolamine (to help the vitamin remain in the blood longer) twice daily—morning and evening—and a 100 mg. tablet of PABA to be taken at noon and at bedtime. He soon observed new pigmentation in the depigmented areas. Within 4 to 8 weeks the milk white areas of vitiligo turned pinkish. In 6 to 16 weeks after therapy was started, small islands of brown pigment were usually noted within the areas of vitiligo. Soon streaks were thrown from these islands and the streaks reached out to join other islands. Eventually the islands disappeared or the repigmentation became complete. The results of the therapy in all 48 patients were termed "striking" after 6 or 7 months.

Dr. Sieve stressed, time and again, the important part diet plays in vitiligo. In his opinion hormonal imbalance can also cause the disease, and contributory factors can be wounds, infections, pressure points and light rays. The problem of vitiligo is more complex than the simple lack of the B vitamin PABA said Sieve. Dietary deficiencies must be corrected, hormonal imbalances righted and local infections cleared up before a single specific vitamin can be expected to have any effect. He also emphasized that the injections to supplement the tablets are essential, because the vitamin alone, taken orally, does not remain in the blood stream for a sufficient length of time to act effectively.

It seems that the B complex, as it appears in brewer's yeast, desiccated liver, wheat germ, and the organ meats, would be effective in preventing vitiligo. This, of course, coupled with a diet complete in other essentials strengthens resistance to most diseases. For those who are plagued with vitiligo, Dr. Sieve's article on his experience points the way to a worthwhile effort against the disease.

Chapter XVII

Warts

The common wart, long a subject for jocular reference to toads, stump water and black cats at midnight in the light of the moon, is actually not a laughing matter. Uncomfortable, unsightly, and often excruciatingly painful (when they are on the bottom of the foot), these pesky growths may be nature's way of signaling trouble ahead.

In a recent study, which promises to have a far-reaching impact on diagnostic procedures, a Philadelphia radiologist Dr. Robert P. Barden, demonstrated that an eruption of warty growths or dermatomyositis might herald a hidden malignancy.

This is not to say that everyone with warts is harboring a pre-cancerous condition. It does mean, however, that the appearance of warts has an important biological significance which it would be wise to investigate.

Why is it, for instance, that warts can sometimes be charmed away by suggestion? Why is it that of all the so-called wart cures, no one method is effective in all cases?

The answer to this therapeutic riddle, says Dr. Daniel Hyman of New York City's Roosevelt Hospital, lies in the viral origin of warts. They disappear when the body's immunologic mechanism is stimulated. The patient himself produces the antibodies. These agents interfere with viral propagation or actually destroy the viruses outright.

Now, what are these host-produced biologic agents and why do some people seem to have an ample supply while others do not? Whatever these still poorly-defined immunologic agents are, their power is enhanced when the body is amply supplied with vitamin A, long recognized as the special guardian of eyes, teeth, bones, skin and soft tissues—the anti-infection vitamin.

Let's review the evidence. What is a wart and what does it have to do with vitamin A? A virus from human warts has been isolated, grown in tissue culture, and then has produced warts after inoculation under the skin of human volunteers. Warts, then, are really benign skin tumors, the only human tumors *proven* to be caused by a virus.

Dr. B. H. Kuhn writing in the *Southern Medical Journal* reports treating 90 patients with various types of warts with vitamin A palmitate in a water dispersible form averaging 25,000 units daily for one week to six months. Cure rates of 50 to 100 per cent were obtained in 79 patients. There were no total failures. Dr. Kuhn suggested in his reports that the vitamin A exerted an *antiviral* action that has specific therapeutic usefulness in the suppression of hyperkeratosis (medical term for "warts").

Some authorities believe that a wart develops where there is a lack of vitamin A in the skin and that introducing the vitamin will bring the skin back to normal. Dr. Marvin Sandler, podiatrist of Allentown, Pennsyl-

[140]

vania, says that he has used an injection of vitamin A on patients with plantar warts on the soles of their feet with excellent results. Another Allentown podiatrist, Dr. Philip LeShay, told us that he prescribes vitamin A systemically in conjunction with other measures in the treatment of warts on the feet.

In the July, 1959, issue of *Clinical Medicine* two researchers reported on the results achieved by 119 physicians who, among them, treated 228 cases of plantar warts with an aqueous solution of vitamin A palmitate. Substantial benefits or complete cures were achieved in 208 of the 228 cases. In only one case did the warts reappear.

In a controlled study of 25 patients at the Jewish hospital of Brooklyn, N.Y., Dr. Joel S. Freeman et al. concluded that the incidence of permanent cures and permanent relief of symptoms is so high, when vitamin A palmitate is used, that it is difficult to justify repeated paring and application of keratolytics and astringents unless vitamin A palmitate has been found to be ineffective. Vitamin A palmitate, Dr. Freeman says, should be tried before resorting to less conservative methods such as surgery, radiation or the stronger caustics.

The fact that both warts and malignancies are on the increase might indicate an increasing inability to manufacture antibodies. Could this inability be related to the increasing depletion of vitamin A in our foods? W. M. Beeson of the Department of Animal Sciences at Purdue University warns that our vitamin A food sources are victims of synthetic nitrogen fertilizers. These compounds act on plants to limit the amount of vitamin A they contain. More than that, the nitrate-loaded foods we eat destroy the vitamin A in our systems. The nitrates make it difficult, and sometimes impossible, for the liver to store vitamin A. The very foods we eat for vitamin A, unless they are organically grown, are likely to contain nitrates absorbed in the field, which inactivate the vitamin A.

Vitamin A is abundant in fats which most calorie-conscious people are avoiding, thus compounding their deficiences. The reduction in intake can be made up, however, with low-calorie foods rich in A, such as pumpkin, carrots, spinach, kale, leaf broccoli, sweet potatoes, apricots, asparagus, parsley, olives, peaches, peas, green and red peppers. Liver of all kinds is rich in vitamin A and lower in calories than muscle meats. Eat these foods and enjoy them.

Chapter XVIII

Drugs and Your Skin

The woman was no longer young. Her children were grown, her first grandchild arrived. But she was slender, vigorous and attractive, and wanted to stay that way. Upon consultation with her doctor during her menopause, she started taking estrogen. (The body's production of this female hormone is drastically reduced when the reproductive years come to a close.)

Aside from estrogen's role in the reproductive cycle, it also helps maintain bone integrity and upright posture, smooth skin, and a full head of hair. Feminine characteristics such as voice pitch and absence of facial hair depend on an estrogen supply. So does a healthy vaginal tract, important to a satisfactory sex life. Female hormones also may play a preventive role in heart health.

Naturally, any woman reaching middle age might consider supplementing the body's dwindling estrogen supply, as the youthful grandmother did. Unfortunately, the very medication she took to maintain her attractiveness caused a disfiguring disease known as *porphyria cutanea tarda*. This metabolic disorder affects the liver and leads to the deposit of the chemical *uroporphyrin* in the skin. The skin becomes photosensitive, increasingly susceptible to damage by heat or

[143]

trauma. Exposed areas of the skin frequently take on a violet-brown pigmentation and develop abnormal hair-growth.

Porphyria cutanea tarda as a side-effect of estrogen therapy was discussed by Drs. Milford Gottlob and Henry H. Roenigk, of the Cleveland Clinic at a meeting of the AMA Section on Dermatology, reported in the November 13, 1969, issue of *Medical Tribune*. These men reviewed 25 cases in the medical literature dating back to 1960, and reported on three additional cases seen in their own clinic.

Though many people take estrogens—and other drugs, for that matter—without suffering a skin reaction, the skin is considered a very reliable barometer for early drug side-effects. Rudolph L. Baer, M.D. and Harriet Harris, M.D. of the department of Dermatology, New York University School of Medicine, attest to the fact, writing in the *Journal of the American Medical Association* (November 20, 1967), "It has long been known that clinically recognizable adverse reactions to drugs are seen more often in the skin than in any other organ or system. . . Because of their frequency and because their visual characteristics alone serve to separate them into a variety of specific types, cutaneous reactions play a particularly important role in the recognization of untoward effects produced by drugs."

It is obvious that a physician must be familiar with characteristic skin changes brought on by bad reactions to particular drugs. But it is also important for the patient to know what a new drug might bring in the way of an allergic skin reaction.

A patient leaves the doctor's office, has the prescription filled. His next appointment is scheduled for a week or two later. If he takes the pills and disregards the itchy red blotches or the strange cluster of blisters that suddenly appear on his skin, he might not live long enough to keep his next appointment.

The reaction associated with each drug is unique. A trained eye can look at a skin change and tell if a specific drug is involved, and how serious the reaction is.

Suppose a patient's skin is breaking out in a kind of acne. If it is sudden, if the skin is not oily and the bumps and pustules are fairly uniform, doctors look for a bromide salt medication, iodides, cortisone compounds, oral contraceptive drugs and certain hormones. When large blisters appear, blisters that contain fluid, an allergic reaction to some arsenic compound is suspected. Other drugs that cause similar eruptions are bromides, barbiturates and sulfonamides.

Because eczema is a common skin problem, its appearance in accompaniment to a streptomycin prescription might easily be misinterpreted. Patches of small, closely gathered blisters or long patches of slight swelling, accompanied by intense itching, can also result from topical application or ingestion of this antibiotic. The same type of eruption results from using mercurials, neomycin, local anesthetics and antihistamines.

Certain anti-convulsants can cause "toxic epidermal necrolysis;" the patient suffering from this reaction sud-

[145]

denly becomes very ill, and the entire skin surface appears scalded and sore. Very large, soft blisters appear; they are easily broken, and leave large sheets of dead tissue which are extremely tender. This sometimes fatal reaction may also follow the use of barbiturates, aminopyrine, phenylbutazone and sulfonamides.

Drugs of the thiazide group and other drug families including antipyrines, penicillin, sulfonamides, bromides, iodides, phenolphthalein, salicylates, cause what the books call "erythema multiforme-like eruptions," definite, sharply separated sores distributed symmetrically over the skin. They fan out from a central lesion to two and three rings in a target pattern. These lesions may be made up of large blisters or small ones. Severe and sometimes fatal forms are generally associated with pneumonia and arthritic cases that call for long-term use of sulfonamides, barbiturates and other drugs.

When skin eruptions are rather flat-topped and purplish, with a distinctive sheen, gold salts (gold sodium thiomalate) may be the cause. A bluish discoloration of the nails is caused by an allergy to amodiaquine. But this often goes unnoticed under fingernail polish.

Redness, swelling and mild scaling from certain drugs shows up only when the user is exposed to sunlight. Photosensitization is characteristic of sulfonamide, sulfonylureas, griseofulvin and chlorpromazine. Externally applied drugs such as bithionol and tetrachlorosalicylanilide can also cause this reaction.

Aspirin is one very commonly used drug that can cause or aggravate skin problems. Those ordinarily subject to hives are likely to suffer even more when

[146]

they take aspirin-containing drugs. Miriam Moore-Robinson and Robert P. Warin, two British physicians, reported that 112 out of 228 experimental patients chronically subject to weals and hives reacted unfavorably to a test dose of aspirin. (*British Medical Journal,* November 4, 1967.) The doctors blamed the salicylic acid.

Fluorides—the chemicals used in fluoridating water supplies—have also been implicated in skin ailments. When a drug company dispenses fluoride tablets it is required by law to warn users never to exceed the recommended dose, which is equal to one quart of fluoridated water. It warns also that even that amount might occasionally cause *eczema, urticaria and atopic dermatitis.*

According to *Prevention* Magazine (November, 1965), a survey of average Milwaukee families showed that twelve out of 100 people reveal, through skin disease, visible signs of fluorine poisoning. In all instances, when fluoridated water was replaced by spring water in the diet of those affected, they were promptly and permanently cured. Here are several of the cases described in the *Prevention* article:

Case No. 1

A 32-year-old mother was in exceptionally good health until she came to fluoridated Milwaukee, ten years ago. Shortly thereafter she developed embarrassing and uncomfortable sores on her face, especially about the mouth; she had chronic sinus colds; her hair became thin; she became an excessive coffee-drinker; but worst of all, she became so tense, that for a time, hospitalization was necessary.

Her doctor recommended that she drink spring water, and almost at once her tension was gone; in about three weeks her skin was normal, and in a couple of months she regained the lost weight and was in perfect health, enjoying life again.

Case No. 2

The subject had no record of skin disease until he came to Milwaukee about eight years ago. Shortly after that he developed a painfully dry throat, and an enormous capacity for drinking water to relieve the dryness; about a gallon a day. His skin became so dry that it peeled; he saw spots before his eyes.

A friend suggested that he try drinking spring water and he found that it quenched his thirst so much better, that almost at once his water consumption returned to normal; his dry throat became comfortable; his skin lost its dryness and his vision was clear again.

Because this man is permanently disabled with emphysema, he was forced to eliminate the expense of spring water. He experienced the same trouble as before after about eight weeks. He resumed drinking spring water once more and the symptoms left him.

Case No. 3

Within three months after this young couple moved to fluoridated Milwaukee from unfluoridated Duluth, they both developed skin disorders and both became extremely nervous. A dermatologist could not relieve their problems.

After about half a year, by chance they moved to unfluoridated Cudahy, and in a short while their skin diseases and nervousness were gone. Until it was called to their attention, the couple never related their trouble to Milwaukee's fluoridated water.

We are not suggesting that all or even most of those who drink fluoridated water will develop skin problems, anymore than most people who wear shoes will develop shoe contact dermatitis. But when a puzzling skin problem exists and fluoridated water is in the picture, a relationship between the two is worth considering.

We really need a deeper undertsanding of what drugs can do for a person and what they can do *to* him. The number of lives saved by drugs is enormous, and we are fortunate to have these weapons against disease. But it is equally true that the excessive, uninformed use of drugs is dangerous. Every patient should approach every drug with suspicion. What is a life-saver for one person may be a killer for another. Know the name of the drug your doctor prescribes. Know what side-effects to expect, particularly on the skin, and keep looking for them.

Chapter XIX

Young Skin Forever

Has there ever been an era like this, when men and women are expected to look 25 even after they've reached 50? To help encourage us to strive for the impossible, cosmetics manufacturers deluge us with "wrinkle-removers" that are guaranteed to erase age-revealing creases on foreheads, cheeks and necks. And every time one company announces a new product along these lines, rival laboratories get busier and busier, trying to outdo each other with "new improved formulas." Just how valuable is all this effort?

Wrinkling and sagging of the skin are primarily due to degeneration of its elastic tissue and loss of fat. Some cosmetics are designed to prevent or curb excessively dry skin; with creams that contain estrogen and progesterone hormones the idea is to produce slight water-logging of the skin.

Though it is known that their effect is only a temporary one, caused by edema (water retention of the tissues) hormone creams are selling briskly. They can make skin look younger for a day or two, and that is enough for the public. Hormone preparations have gained further status through the use of estrogen by some doctors to delay menopause in women. The theory is this: if estrogen levels that normally decrease

[150]

in menopause are maintained artificially, the onset of wrinkly skin, sagging breasts, arthritis, heart disease and diabetes is delayed.

Of course, this idea appeals to women, but no one knows what the adverse effects will be. We do know that tampering with the delicate hormonal balance can cause serious reactions, including the possible development of cancer. One gynecologist stated, "We've had numerous patients with hysterectomies and bad hot flashes. We give them estrogens. A couple of them blew up with cancer of the breast." He added that estrogen may not have been the direct cause of the cancer, but it does appear to be a cancer stimulant.

The International Institute for Age Therapy suggested that a patient who has extended treatment with estrogen may have such serious adverse reactions as ovarian seizure, arterial thrombosis, retinal blindness, edema, varicose veins or weight gain. If diuretics are prescribed to help release the water, their prolonged use causes a variety of metabolic disorders.

That such judgments do not seem to dampen the enthusiasm of cosmetics companies for hormone creams is to be expected. But it seems that too many of the beautifying methods women are willing and eager to try are dangerous, fail completely, or at best, produce only short-term results. Even face lifts must be periodically redone at considerable cost in time and money. A lifetime of good habits can help prevent menopausal disorders that frighten so many women into thinking they need hormone supplements or injections.

Cosmetics cover; they do not cure. If you must use

[151]

cosmetics, choose a type made from natural products. It is about time that we all learned to stay away from youth preparations that contain coal tars, hormones and other substances whose effects we cannot possibly know.

There may be a safe answer to aging skin in the recent discovery of Benjamin S. Frank, M.D. The New York doctor seems to have come up with a natural, and apparently harmless, type of skin cream that is different in character and effect from other cosmetics.

Dr. Frank has prescribed his newly developed cream for more than 100 patients, ranging in age from 21 to 84. While the effect varies somewhat from one person to another, he has not found a single patient on whose skin the cream did not have some noticeable rejuvenating effect.

"Without any other medication given," he said, "this cream applied nightly to the whole face reduced lines and wrinkles, including the depths of the nasal labial folds (the lines from the nostrils to the corners of the mouth) and reduced crows feet around the eyes and deeper wrinkles in the forehead very noticeably."

And what is the remarkable material that can have such an incredible effect on the appearance of the face? It is simply yeast—a strain of yeast closely related to brewer's yeast but selected because it is even richer than brewer's yeast in nucleic acid. The yeast is dissolved in water, which frees its considerable natural content of nucleic acid, and the resulting fluid is mixed into a cold cream base.

Dr. Frank insists that his nucleic acid cream is *not* a

[152]

wrinkle cream, and not a cosmetic preparation. "I'm really not even interested in wrinkles," he says, "It's the reversal of aging that I'm working on and the only reason I even developed this cream was because so many of my patients are foolishly in a greater hurry to get rid of the visible appearance of aging—the wrinkles and bags and sometimes brown spots—than they are to eliminate the more basic and serious effects that aging can have on a person. It's just a peculiarity of human nature that a woman will be more anxious to look ten years younger than she is to reduce her high blood pressure."

Dr. Frank is more interested in the blood pressure, the heart, the bones and vital capacity, as well as other organs and functions that tend to degenerate as age advances. Nucleic acids, DNA and RNA, are the actual materials that control the ability of the individual body cell to keep replicating itself and reproducing its inherited patterns. Dr. Frank believes that the nucleic acids themselves can age for lack of sufficient fresh material with which to reproduce themselves. In so aging, he theorized, these strands of acid found within the cell nucleus would either have their information blurred so that the cell would not work and reproduce itself as accurately, or else they would completely lose their information and the cell would die.

What is it that permits the skin on the back of an aged hand to become shiny, wrinkled, spotted and brittle? The cells which contain the blueprint for the formation of that hand are tired, worn and no longer able to maintain the pattern they inherited.

[153]

In Dr. Frank's opinion, the problem of maintaining youthfulness is the problem of finding ways to help your body's DNA and RNA renew themselves and keep their patterns of genetic information as clean and fresh as a new etching.

Reduced to its essence, he considers it the problem of supplying the body from external sources with enough viable nucleic acids and with the other nutrients these nucleic acids require to be properly metabolized. Given such nutrition, he believes, the nucleic acids themselves stay younger longer, and this is reflected in the tissues they control.

One regime used by Dr. Frank included large doses of yeast RNA on the order of 5 to 10 grains of RNA taken one, two or three times weekly with B-complex capsules taken daily with the noon meal. The most striking effects were observed on the skin of the face. The higher the dosage, the more rapidly these effects occurred: alteration in skin aspect toward a healthier, rosier looking skin and simultaneously an apparent smoothing of the skin of the face, without any change yet in wrinkles and lines. These early effects occurred within the first or second week of treatment, usually within the first week. After one or two months of treatment, sometimes earlier, not only did the smoothness and color of the skin improve, but lines and wrinkles began to diminish.

The wrinkles in the forehead were often the first to decrease in depth. The lines around the eyes took longer to decrease in depth. Though there was not a total disappearance of any wrinkles or lines, there was

[154]

in a large majority of cases a distinctly noticeable decrease in their depth.

As the wrinkles decreased, skin tightness and the moistness of the skin increased. These are the advertised, but seldom achieved, effects of expensive facial creams.

Dr. Frank found it inadvisable to administer very large doses of nucleic acid orally. The effect was like that of an unusually high protein diet—beneficial to most people, yet occasionally resulting in levels of uric acid high enough to pose a threat to the kidneys. It was partly for this reason that he reduced the oral dosage and developed this skin cream as a substitute. In doing so, he may have formulated the treatment for aging skin that has been sought through history.

Chapter XX

Cosmetics

Aided by large scale advertising campaigns, cosmetics are snapped up as fast as they appear on the market. Labels that promise magic, easily lure teenagers and matrons alike. Common sense tells us that the products cannot possibly match the claims, yet it's hard to resist lavish advertising that assures a "new" you.

Every year the public spends between 6 and 8 billion dollars on cosmetics, and this amount is growing. For the beauty industry the future looks bright; for consumers the outlook could be grim.

In October, 1967, the A.M.A. and the Society of Toxicology co-sponsored a symposium on *The Evaluation of Cosmetics* in Washington, D.C. One of the speakers at that meeting, Dr. Paul Lazar of Northwestern University Medical School, showed actual slides of men and women whose arms, backs, faces and legs had been disfigured by cosmetic products used every day by most people.

Some of the victims Lazar discussed had large red blots over parts of their body. Others were covered with large scabs or scales.

Almost all the cases were photodermatoses—chemical reactions between particular cosmetics and the ultraviolet rays from the sun. Who are the people who have these reactions? How rare are they? Science cannot answer those questions. But one thing is quite obvious—at least to the dermatologists who were at the Washington meeting—the number of people becoming susceptible to photoallergic reactions is definitely on the increase.

The indelible dyes in lipstick, for example, act as photosensitizers which can produce swelling when the lips are exposed to the sun. These dyes (used to make lipsticks smear-proof) combine with the skin of the lips and cause cracking, drying and peeling, swelling, puffiness and tenderness. There are even lipsticks that don't color—their sole purpose is to provide a moist look. These extras increase the chances of reaction. And some of the lipstick applied so lavishly throughout the day is inevitably swallowed or absorbed through the skin. Who knows what the cumulative effect will be?

Beauty, once called the reflection of the soul, is now established as an item you can buy at the cosmetics counter. American women of every age smear their faces with countless concoctions, and dye their hair to match their moods, their outfits or their neighbors. To look younger, they plaster over the wrinkles; to look alluring, they add eyelashes, and, to look "natural" they blend endless varieties of foundations, blushers, eye shadows and lipsticks. Any magazine that caters to women describes, at regular intervals, how to achieve the latest cosmetic "look." What the maga-

[157]

zines don't report is that the price of the look may be bad skin.

As the types of available cosmetics increase, so do the instances of bad reactions to the ingredients in them. "Women with skin or respiratory symptoms should be aware of the fact that their problems can be caused or aggravated by the cosmetics they use," says Dr. S. J. Taub, writing in *The Eye, Ear, Nose and Throat Monthly* (Volume 44, August 1965). For virtually every cosmetic preparation, there is someone who will experience an unfavorable reaction to it.

With any inflammation of the skin (dermatitis) due to cosmetics, the major problem is a sensitizer—an agent which appears innocuous when it is first applied, but gradually stimulates an allergic reaction.

There are plenty of sensitizers, and even very small amounts of the wrong chemical can produce a dermatitis in the right person. The reaction may appear as a rash, accompanied by itchiness, swelling, dryness, skin cracking or nasal irritation similar to hay fever or a cold.

Dr. James W. Burks, writing in the *Journal of the Southern Medical Association* (October, 1962) warned that even if the chemicals in a cosmetic are free of irritants at the time of packaging, "they may deteriorate with time or become altered by contact with containers, exposure to light, or other reactive substances, and thus act as primary irritants when used."

Consider the variety of beauty products in use and you get some idea of the problem cosmetic reactions present. The many types of dyeing preparations represent big trouble all by themselves, especially since more women than ever before are changing their hair color. One dye in particular, paraphenylenediamine, has a high sensitizing potential. Dr. Burks says: "Reactions to this dye have been not only frequent, but the most severe of all reactions to cosmetics." He calls the reaction "explosive!"—an initial tightness of the scalp is soon followed by painful tenderness and later a weeping, acute inflammation.

There is no sidestepping the fact that hair dyes, sprays and waving lotions cause a wide variety of injuries. When the original Food, Drug and Cosmetic Act was created in 1938, Congress, convinced of the danger of the coal-tar dyes, forbade their use in cosmetics, in spite of stiff pressure from industry groups.

One industry group, the hair dye manufacturers, refused to accept the order. They insisted that there was no way to make a satisfactory product without the forbidden ingredients. The legislature was warned that if the coal-tar dyes were not reinstated, women from all over the country would march on the Capitol in rage.

The lawmakers gave-in. Coal-tar would be permitted in hair dyes, but the label must warn of danger to the eyes; the subject must be tested for any sensitivity to ingredients. The result is that a significant number of women have been injured by the dyes. Most never see the label, since the dyes are used primarily by beauticians. And virtually no one is ever tested for sensitivity before use.

About 24 per cent of all cosmetics complaints made today are attributed to hair dyes. The injuries range from mild skin irritation on the scalp to serious rash, fever, pustules and infection. According to an FDA spokesman, "The person who suffers a severe reaction is seriously ill and may require hospitalization followed by medical treatment for months."

The industry figures show that 20 million to 30 million women dye their hair—and more and more men are doing so. As product use continues to grow, so do the adverse reactions.

The darker dyes require paradiaminobenzenes and aminophenols, two powerful compounds which are part of the chemical group known as aniline dyes. *Clinical Toxicology of Commercial Products* (published by Williams and Wilkins) remarks: "Many poisonings are reported each year from exposure to aniline and related substances . . ." Blood changes, kidney and liver problems are not unusual consequences of aniline poisonings. Occasionally, the injured lady takes action.

An Oklahoma cosmetics retailer was found liable for a customer's matted and lost hair caused by a hair spray.

In California, a beautician was found negligent in applying "Miss Clairol" hair bleach without giving the costumer a "patch test" for sensitivity. (The maker of the bleach, Clairol, Inc., has sued a number of discount stores for selling *Miss Clairol Hair Color Bath,* intended for beauty parlor use only, without the warnings given to beauticians. The firm said that some "hypersensitive" persons "may be left with very unhappy

[160]

results" and implied that a beautician would protect a customer against such results.)

Cosmetics intended for fingernails can make trouble just as the hair products do—and bad reactions are not limited to the fingers. Fingernail cosmetics have been responsible for damage to eyes, face, neck and other parts of the body—even when they were used as intended!

One woman won't forget her experience with a fingernail hardener. She applied it to her nails and some hours later noticed that they were turning blue. By the next morning, her fingers were bleeding, and the pain was so excruciating that the woman had to be given heavy doses of pain killers.

Nail polishes which contain resins (and almost all of them do) cause trouble in some unexpected places. Despite the fact that chemicals are applied to the fingernails, eruptions are most common on those parts of the body habitually touched by the fingers—such as the face, ears, neck and eyelids. The lacquer has even caused dermatitis in the children and spouse of the person wearing the polish.

Some cosmetics, such as hair removers, are by their very nature potentially injurious to the skin. Their formulas include salts of thioglycolic acid and a few contain sulfides, particularly strontium sulfide, all of which can produce strong irritation. Reactions are especially likely to occur if the dipilatory remains on the skin too long, or if it's applied to sensitive areas such as the underarms.

Face creams cause more than their share of trouble,

[161]

since their formulas are often extremely complex. Lanolin, a natural oil secreted from the sebaceous glands of sheep, is a popular but allergenic face cream ingredient. It can produce severe redness, itching and blotchy skin spots.

Walter F. Edmundson, M.D., and associates reported in *Industrial Medicine and Surgery* (December, 1967) that the lanolin you rub on your face might be contaminated with harmful pesticides. When sheep are treated with these chemicals the animals' natural oils and fats tend to absorb them. When random samples of lipsticks, hair dressings, eyeshadow, creams, lotions and baby oils containing lanolin are analyzed DDT shows up in appreciable amounts.

When all other make-up has been applied, a woman adds the finishing touch—a few drops of her favorite scent. Perfume has an extraordinary capacity for causing allergic complications. Most commercial fragrances are complicated mixtures which usually include several synthetic materials. Dr. Burks says: "The complexity of the problem is apparent from the fact that there are approximately 5,000 odoriferous substances in use today," and "the essential perfume oils used in cosmetics contain 50 or more basic components." Any of the perfumed powders, bath soaps, and deodorants might cause reactions due to these oils. Dr. Taub estimates that "one woman in ten has either a respiratory or skin allergy to perfumes and colognes."

Most cosmetics present another danger area for consumers. Though the claim is seldom made, the implication is that medicated lipsticks, powders, rouges, etc., are perfectly safe to use.

However—"Incorporation of pharmacologically active ingredients into cosmetics which are sold across the counter is objectionable because no absorbable drug should be given without control of dosage," according to Stephen Rothman, M.D., a dermatologist of the Department of Medicine of the University of Chicago, in an address to a recent meeting of the Society of Cosmetic Chemists. Further expressing his opposition to the concept of drugs in cosmetics, he said:

"Cosmetics are being sold across the counter; therefore, there is no limit to the absolute dose. No drug has been shown so far to have no percutaneous (through the skin) absorption at all . . . There is no drug which sooner or later would not cause any harm if given without any restriction of the dosage . . ."

But if the unlimited use of any drug can be dangerous what drugs are used in medicated cosmetics and how dangerous are they?

Many acne lotions on the market contain resorcin, a drug that can have an adverse effect on latent kidney disorders.

Rejuvenating skin creams are generally rich in estrogenic hormones. As far back as 1952, the *AMA Journal* reported that such hormones are easily absorbed through the skin. They are known to cause irregular menstrual staining, and could promote the development of ovarian cancer. Such hormones affect the appearance of the skin by binding water in the tissues and

[163]

causing a swelling that seems to smooth wrinkles. Most of the skin creams that claim to be good for boils, pimples and acne, contain antibiotics. For a long while penicillin was a common ingredient, but the number of sensitized people who suffered strong allergic reactions grew so great that the drug had to be discontinued. Now other antibiotics, tyrothricin, bacitracin, polymyxin B and neomycin sulfate, are substituted. Safe? They are drugs and it is Dr. Rothman's judgment that any drug will cause harm if used long enough.

An area of serious concern in any discussion of cosmetics is their relation to cancer. Eugene J. Van Scott, M.D., speaking at the cosmetics conference mentioned early in this chapter, said "We have never shown that cosmetics do not cause cancer . . . Certainly in the past century both known and unknown carcinogenic substances have appeared in cosmetics formulas." And some, he said, are used even today.

Van Scott told his audience that cosmetics are applied to the lips, the mucous tissues, and are inhaled. Known cancer-causers, when they enter the body, may not affect the tissues through which they enter, he warned, but may produce a cancer in a distant tissue or organ.

The prevailing situation was summarized in the January 1, 1968 issue of *The Nation*: "Although the cosmetic industry protests that the products of the 1930's which contained caustic chemicals and poisons are gone, the 1938 legislation hasn't prevented such periodic shockers as a hair straightener that used lye, a hair dryer with carbon tetrachloride (a potent liver poison) and a cleansing cream colored with 'butter yellow,' a known cancer-producing chemical. Neither did it prevent wholesale injuries by a number of shampoos, nail-base polishes, plastic nails and a permanent wave neutralizer."

Back in 1961, Dr. Irvin Kerlan, director of the Research and Reference Branch of the FDA's Bureau of Medicine, said, "It is fair to add that we (at FDA) have given only minimum attention to cosmetics as a class because of a limited staff." At the 1968 Washington meeting Associate Commissioner Kirk admitted that things still had not changed.

Of the thousands made, only five batches of cosmetic products were seized in 1970: three because of bacterial contamination, one because of misbranding, and one because the product, a deodorant, contained glass particles.

A recent report from Saint Vincent Hospital in Worcester, Massachusetts, indicates that, even where FDA has the power to regulate against cosmetics, it is falling down on the job. Of twenty-six brands of hand lotion examined at the hospital, four were found to be contaminated with bacteria.

Since 1953, Rep. Leonor K. Sullivan (D-Mo) has been doing everything in her power to get a bill through Congress that would give the Food and Drug Administration the responsibility of making sure that all ingredients in a cosmetic are safe. But every one of her proposals has failed. In 1966 Rep. Sullivan said, "The consumer is being used as a guinea pig on

[165]

each new cosmetic item. If enough consumers get hurt
—burned or scalped or disfigured or scarred or infected from a new untested cosmetic—the government
eventually hears about it and moves against the product and takes it off the market. But, oh, the agony in
the meantime!"

Mrs. Sullivan is determined to continue introducing
protective legislation every year, though chances for
success are minimal. Opposition comes not only from
the incredibly powerful Toilet Goods Association and
the cosmetics industry lobby, but from the FDA!

At the Washington Cosmetics conference, Kirk
promised that there will be significant legislation introduced in Congress that *may* extend FDA jurisdiction
over toiletry and cosmetics products, *"if the FDA and
the industry can reach agreement* on what the bill
ought to be." The Sullivan bill is aimed four-square at
protecting the health of the consumer. It appears that
the FDA/industry bill, if any, will be framed to protect the cosmetics industry from government control.

What Mrs. Sullivan is after—and what is vitally
needed for the protection of the consumer—is preclear-
ance of all new cosmetic products. As Rudolph L.
Baer, M.D., of the N.Y.U. School of Medicine points
out, side-effects of an ingredient in cosmetics are very
difficult to track down once the product reaches the
marketplace. Unlike prescription drugs, no records are
kept of their sale and user-reaction. And, says Baer,
"Not only are there very few publications appearing
in ethical medical journals to indicate that new ingredients have been added to, or used in, cosmetics, but

[166]

for reasons which are inherent in the practices of the cosmetic industry, it is sometimes difficult for physicians to obtain pertinent information from the manufacturers."

What it boils down to is an official attitude that cosmetics are innocent until proven guilty. That is as potentially dangerous an idea with cosmetics as it is with drugs. Dr. Van Scott, who spoke at the Washington Conference, said at the meeting, "Cosmetics are secondary to life. They are not necessary for survival. And they are not necessary for reproduction. It's time we did some monitoring of the effects these chemicals are having on humans. Use of materials in cosmetics should be limited to those of known safety."

Will we ever get a good law? Ultimately, the consumer sends the lawmakers to Washington. Letters and personal visits can pressure representatives to vote for *meaningful* cosmetics laws.

In the meantime, the best guarantee of a beautiful skin is good health. Watch your diet and make sure it supplies every vitamin and mineral in sufficient amounts; exercise and get proper rest. You will see your skin, like the rest of you, come alive with vitality and beauty.

When you do use cosmetics, stick to the natural ones that contain neither drugs nor chemicals. They won't treat skin diseases or rejuvenate. But neither will they do any harm.

Chapter XXI

Hair

Hair is considered woman's crowning glory and a sign of virility in men. Tales of Rapunzel and Samson serve as reminders of its romantic connotations. Small wonder that women are willing to try almost anything to enhance the appearance of their tresses. A lady not blessed with naturally-curly hair turns to permanent waving. If her natural color isn't right, a bottle of hair dye will quickly change it. Backcombing, to make hair look thicker than it is, has become a common practice. As a result of this kind of tampering, baldness has become more prevalent; dull, lifeless hair (the opposite of the desired effect) is the rule, not the exception.

The low-protein, high-carbohydrate diet that is a way of life today compounds the problem. Your hair is 97 percent protein and three percent minerals and ash. So it's not surprising that a diet rich in protein, along with other nutrients, is essential to keeping it healthy.

Normal nutritional equilibrium for the hair must include phosphoric acid, calcium, vitamin B 12 and pantothenic acid. *The Canadian Medical Association Journal* (June 26, 1965) made special mention of deficiencies of riboflavin and vitamin A as inhibitors of hair growth. Harold H. Perlenfein, of the Lee Foundation of Nutritional Research, says a deficiency of unsaturated fatty acids can be the cause of falling hair. But protein is the most critical and most often lacking ingredient of healthy hair.

Hair is naturally acid-balanced. On an acid-alkaline scale of 14 (acid is 1, alkaline 14, 7 is neutral) hair should register between 4.5 and 4.7. To have really healthy hair, this delicate balance must be maintained. Since most hair products sold today are alkaline, hair is constantly being pushed to the wrong end of the scale.

How can you determine whether your favorite shampoo is acidic or (as is most likely the case) alkaline? The procedure is amazingly simple. From any drug store, purchase a package of Nitrazine pH paper. This comes with a color-keyed scale. Simply put the end of the paper in the solution you want to test and match the resulting color to the color scale to find out just how acidic or alkaline the product is.

Don't bother to make this test on permanent wave solution or hair dye. These are all alkaline by definition. There is no way of using them without damaging your hair to some extent, no matter what your beautician may tell you. If skillfully used, some of these products are less harmful than others, but they all draw vitality from the hair leaving it dull and lifeless looking.

If a hair product's label says "organic" or "natural," the item is worth special consideration. But labels can be misleading. Opportunists sometimes abuse and misuse these terms deliberately. It is currently popular to

[169]

feature protein as an ingredient. This sounds good, and indeed it is if the product contains between 40 and 50 percent protein. Shampoos of this type have been known to increase tensile strength as much as 75 percent in one washing. However, most products which boast about their protein content contain no more than one percent—just enough to meet legal requirements, but not enough to do any good. When considering a shampoo, setting lotion, or rinse that advertises its "protein" content, write to the manufacturer and ask what percentage of protein is in his product. If it's 40 to 50 percent buy it; if not, keep shopping for another shampoo.

Be selective about the comb you use. The metal combs and plastic combs have sharp edges which damage the delicate hair shaft. The best choice is a hard rubber comb with blunt teeth. Your brush should be made of natural bristles. Many people have ruined their hair by brushing it with synthetic bristles.

A healthy head of hair depends on a healthy scalp. Each hair grows in a tiny indentation in the skin, called a follicle, at the base of which is tissue containing blood vessels that supply food to the hair. Hair does not have "roots." What appears as a small bulb on the end of a hair you pull out is actually the lining of the follicle in which the hair was growing. The hair itself contains no nerves. A tiny muscle is attached to the follicle which responds instantly and automatically to the stimulation of fright or cold, causing one's hair to "stand on end" or causing "goose flesh."

The pigment which gives hair its color is located in

the layer of the hair, called the cortex. As hair grows, the old hair moves up the inside of the follicle, depositing a column of cells behind it, which will form the new hair. So long as old hairs continue to deposit this column of cells, the rate of hair growth will keep pace with the rate of hair loss.

Hair grows at the rate of approximately one inch in six weeks. It grows more rapidly in summer than in winter and grows fastest between the age of 35 and 60—the very age when baldness in some individuals is most common!

When hair is healthy, the rate of replacement keeps abreast of the rate of loss. But once an old hair leaves its follicle, without depositing the vital growing nucleus, there will be no new hair to replace it.

When we think of hair problems, dandruff is one of the first to come to mind. Dandruff is the result of the outermost layers of the scalp's skin scaling off, a process that goes on with the skin all over the body. It is more obvious on the head and hair because the scales tend to accumulate and show up in contrast to dark hair or dark clothing. This "simple dandruff" leaves no redness or inflammation of the scalp and causes no loss of hair. "Aggravated dandruff," however, is frequently a sign of imminent baldness, since the surface of the scalp is involved, becoming moist and reddened under the scales. Though both the "simple" and "aggravated" types of dandruff affect only the outermost layers of the scalp, "aggravated" conditions can lead to seborrhea, a disease that shows up in the sebaceous glands. Known also as "pathological dan-

[171]

druff," the disease occurs when the quantity of oil from these sebaceous glands is in excess of the means nature provides for drainage.

To prevent dandruff, Dr. Herman Goodman, in his book, *Your Hair,* urges frequent washing of comb and brush with soap and water, and discourages the use of stinging antiseptic "tonics." Since the disease is apparently a concomitant of civilization, he concludes that its appearance tends to coincide with rundown health. As dietary precautions against such "civilization diseases," he advises limiting sugars and starches; including more vegetables, both cooked and raw, in the diet; and drinking eight glasses of water daily.

Shampoo at least once a week if the scalp is normal, to keep the hair clean, healthy and free of dandruff. Oily scalps should be washed oftener. Dr. Goodman believes hard water should not be used for shampoos, since it makes soaps insoluble, deprives them of the ability to cleanse, and causes them to adhere to the hair. He warns against shampoos that contain a large quantity of coconut oil because it tends to irritate the scalp. Lemon and vinegar rinses are recommended by him because they restore the normal acidity to an adult's scalp, which is in an alkaline state immediately after shampooing. (Lemon juice should always be diluted, because it makes the hair too acidic when used full strength.)

We have only touched upon another problem which concerns many people—baldness. To a man, the sight of a hairbrush full of lost hairs is cause for concern, perhaps reflection on the passing years; for a woman

[172]

it's a ticket to hysteria. Dermatologist Howard T. Behrman, M.D., of New York Medical College said it: "All women tend to become hysterical and some psychotic at the thought of impending baldness."

Experts estimate that currently one out of three women has a hair loss problem, and the statistics are going up.

The surest evidence that something is wrong with the American woman's hair comes from the drug industry's records of increased sales for products to treat damaged hair. Unfortunately, many of these so-called remedies only further the damage. In a survey conducted a few years ago by a prominent shampoo manufacturer, 89 percent of the women who answered complained of having one or more hair care problems, a figure that was up 5 percent from the preceding year's survey. No wonder hair from American women is not in great demand for wigs, toupees, etc. Most sought after is the hair of middle and southern European women, especially farm women. Their hair is rich and thick, well textured and has a high luster. Their diets are generally simpler than those of American women and they don't have ready access to fancy hair products.

Unlike male baldness, baldness in women apparently has little connection with age. Victor Witten, M.D., one of the authors of a definitive paper on baldness for the AMA's *Book of Health,* found that 40 percent of the women suffering from unexplained baldness were between 26 and 46 years of age. But

[173]

some of the others were teenagers, and some were over 60.

The good side, if there is a good side, is that the type of baldness prevalent among females is never the shiny-domed, clean-sweep type that afflicts many men. Known as diffuse alopecia, the thinning may get progressively worse, but the loss will stop eventually. In Dr. Behrman's words, "The woman must simply get used to a thinner crop. She'll have enough to set adequately and it will look pretty good." Some comfort, but not much.

What better source for the real story on why so much goes wrong with so many women's hair than the *Journal of the American Medical Women's Association?* In the June, 1966 issue, Dr. Norman Orentreich indicted the chemicals brought into contact with the hair for cosmetic reasons. "Such preparations usually affect only the hair shaft and cause hair to become fragile and break. But, if improperly compounded or applied, some cosmetic chemicals may irritate the underlying or adjacent scalp." As for permanent wave solutions, the AMA has stated that these chemicals can act as a depilatory (hair remover) when left on the scalp too long.

Several London researchers explored the cause of hair loss in women and their analysis of 95 baldness cases showed that nearly half were associated with the use of harsh hair cosmetics. Dr. Suzanne Alexander said (*Worldwide Abstracts,* March-April, 1966), 21 of the patients were bald due to hair straighteners. Hair dressing accidents, due to permanent waving, bleaching and chemicals, occurred in three patients; 15 were bald because of the hair rollers they used. Regrowth occurred in most of these women when they stopped using whatever caused the baldness.

Drugs and poisons are named by Dr. Orentreich in the *JAMWA* for their bad effect on hair. "The antimetabolites, coming into increasing prominence for the treatment of such varied conditions as leukemias and lymphomas, choriocarcinoma, the so-called auto-immune states, and psoriasis, interfere with cell division specifically and thus commonly damage the mitotically highly active hair matrix."

The AMA Committee on Cosmetics said in 1963 that increased exposure to synthetic detergents, additives in commercial shampoos, increased use of antibiotics in the diets of meat animals, air pollution, crop sprays and radioactive fallout are all threats to human hair.

Treating women with male hormones, a medical practice that has become common in recent years, may give rise to severe baldness, Edwin Sidi and Mme. Bourgeois-Spinasse wrote in *Press Medicale,* (66/79). They found the first warning to be an oily scalp, with hairs sticking together. These hairs give way at the slightest pull of a comb or brush.

More than a decade ago, Eugene Foldes linked salt intake with baldness by counting the number of hairs which came out of the scalp each day under experimental conditions in a man who was becoming bald on top. He found the loss of hair fairly constant until the subject began two days or more of unrestricted salt

[175]

intake. His article in *Acta. Med. Scandinav.* (volume 159, 1957) stated that the loss was always significantly increased with heavy salt intake.

Anyone with a hair problem will tell you, "Everybody has a cure!" Like hiccups. Some of the ideas are old wives' tales and far out stunts that no one really expects will work. But there are reasonable, effective preventives against baldness.

First of all, before she does anything drastic, a lady whose scalp is starting to show should check on whether she isn't suffering from any one of a number of temporary types of baldness. Certain diseases with high fever, pregnancy and menopause cause some women to lose their hair. Usually, a little patience and forbearance will see the return of the original crop.

Another remediable kind of baldness is due to emotional tension. Along these lines, Dr. William J. Bryan, Jr., of Tulane University found to his amazement that hypnosis can reverse hair loss. Hypnotized for sinus trouble, he grew a full head of hair as a side effect! The American Institute of Hypnosis said, "The Tulane physician age-regressed under medical hypnosis to correct the psychological cause of sinus trouble and proved that if hair follicles are still alive the pituitary gland can send hair growing hormones to the scalp or other parts of the body."

Good nutrition is still the basic ingredient for the health and maintenance of a good head of hair, and if one would avoid baldness, this is the place to start.

[176]

Your hair is only as healthy as you are. Nourish it and take care of it as you do any other part of your body. If you abuse your health, you can expect things to go wrong with your hair.

Chapter XXII

The Natural Beauty Plan

The formula for beautiful skin is really a simple one: good nutrition plus planned exercise plus cleanliness plus sufficient sleep. There are beauty techniques, of course, that go along with the above, but for one who is concerned enough to carry out the basic formula, additional skin care becomes a matter of enjoyment.

Since nutrition can make or break the above formula for a healthy skin, examine your individual nutritional needs. Keep the phrase "balanced nutrition" in mind. It is not one magical food but overall diet that affects beauty.

With a carefully chosen, varied diet, you can maintain the vigor of your body at its highest level, and you can help repair damages to your appearance due to neglect in the past.

Beauty begins in the kitchen. What takes place there today determines your complexion tomorrow. The quality of food, the method of preparation and your overall plan of nourishment all have a part in influencing your health and beauty.

The value of exercise is exactly the same to the skin as it is to other body organs. It stimulates hormonal secretions, increases metabolism, feeds needed blood to the tissues and firms muscles. This is true of any general exercise such as brisk walking, jogging, swimming or cycling. Make it a point to include such exercises in your daily schedule. But beyond that, there are specific exercises for the face—the most obvious skin tissue of all.

The value of facial exercises is epitomized by Marjorie Craig, exercise supervisor at the Elizabeth Arden salon in New York City. She is one of those rare women who has an almost incredible ability to maintain her appearance of youth and beauty.

Miss Craig believes that facial aging is caused by sagging skin and weak underlying muscles. Wrinkling of the forehead, crow's feet at the corners of the eyes, creases between the eyebrows, and deep furrows on the cheeks all result from disuse or misuse of the facial muscles.

The most common exercises used to improve the strength of the facial muscles are the isometric ones, the same type used since the turn of the century to build up arms, legs, and trunks. These exercises can help to smooth the wrinkles around the eyes, nose and forehead, erase a double chin, or minimize that jowly look or the drawn, even haggard appearance that often accompanies aging.

What are isometrics? Simply stated, they're exercises which contract body muscles without moving the body parts involved. Muscles are tensed against immovable objects or contracted by holding two joints rigid and tensing the muscles between them. (In contrast, isotonic exercises—the kind used in doing push-

[179]

ups and other general calisthenics—stretch the muscles and move body parts.)

Isometric exercises affect only the voluntary muscles —that is, they do not apply to the internal muscles of the heart, blood vessels and intestines. For that reason, any exercise program based on isometrics should also include isotonic exercises to benefit the respiratory and circulatory systems.

Laboratory experiments have shown that when muscles are tensed to two-thirds of their maximum contraction for 6 to 10 seconds each day, their strength will increase considerably. Although medical literature lacks the before-and-after measurements proving that isometrics really work on the face, advocates of facial exercise say there is every reason to believe facial muscles react as other body muscles do.

Although all of the facial muscles are under voluntary control, few people are used to thinking about using this control deliberately, and particularly about how to contract one muscle or group of muscles without using many others at the same time. It does require considerable concentration and effort in front of a mirror to learn to contract only the desired muscles, while keeping the others relaxed.

Miss Craig stresses the fact that these exercises must be done slowly. A muscle will not develop strength in an isometric contraction, which is essentially what these exercises are, unless the contraction is maintained for a certain period of time. There is no general agreement as to how long, but it seems doubtful if contractions held for less than six seconds are effective.

[180]

Here is a group of facial exercises heralded by a number of fitness authorities.

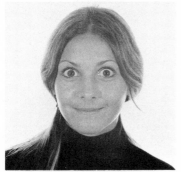

Eyes—To erase crow's feet and strengthen muscles behind the eyes, Clara E. Patterson tells you to: open your eyes as wide as possible, first looking up, then down, then to the left, and to the right. Hold each position for a slow count of six.

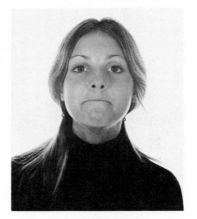

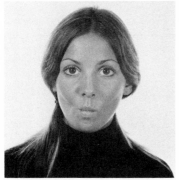

Cheeks—To reduce overly full cheeks follow this exercise by Debbie Drake: Close mouth and space teeth slightly apart, now suck cheeks between your teeth. Relax and repeat several times.

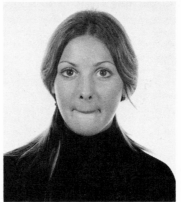

Nose—Marjorie Craig's "Nose Wrinkler" fills in furrows between nose and cheeks. Slightly open mouth and flare out nostrils as you wrinkle up nose, causing upper lip to draw up. Now concentrate on moving upper lip down, which will also lower nose. Repeat exercise 5 times.

[181]

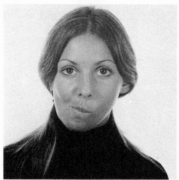

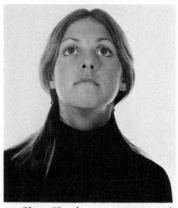

Mouth—Firm the muscles of the mouth, chin, and cheeks with these two exercises by Sara Mildred Strauss. Open mouth wide then bring lips together as to kiss. Repeat slowly ten times. With lips puckered move lips in a circle from left to right, then from right to left. Repeat eight times for each side.

Chin—Here's an exercise offered by Gunilla Knutson to firm the chin line: With your head thrown back, try to bite an imaginary apple with only your lower lip. If properly done, both neck and chin muscles will pull. Repeat 15 times.

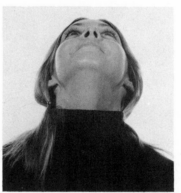

Neck—To strengthen neck muscles and release tension, Jack La-Lanne advises you to: Pull your head back far enough to look at the ceiling, then contract neck muscles. Relax and repeat several times.

An essential part of the formula for beautiful skin is cleanliness—and sometimes that may mean cleansing the skin of skin.

The four layers of the skin are constantly growing and renewing themselves. The epidermis, or outer layer, should be flexible and elastic, to accommodate the needs of your body. It is this layer that constantly flakes off, being renewed by the layers underneath. To ignore this, to be unaware of the need for a little friction occasionally to remove the dead, flaked-off cells, is to invite trouble in the form of clogged and enlarged pores and lifeless looking skin that cannot breathe.

Many methods and preparations have been created to do this job. Of course, the one you choose must be gentle. Harsh treatments or rough preparations can damage your skin.

First study your skin in a magnifying mirror to determine its condition. For lifeless, unhealthy-looking skin, perhaps a complexion brush is in order. This little wonder will stimulate your skin even as it removes the dead cells. It cleanses deep enough to unclog the pores, renewing their ability to breathe and sustain their own cleanliness.

Even more effective and stronger than the complexion brush is the following preparation. Use it once a week without fail.

Bring a couple of cups of water to boil in an immaculate basin. Never use aluminum for this preparation. Drop in one papaya mint teabag, or just a plain papaya teabag without the mint, if you prefer. Allow the tea to simmer a bit, remove from the fire and steep. If you are impatient to get on with it, add a bit of cold water and then squeeze out the tea bag and dispose of it. Take a white, terry washcloth and dip it into the brew, wring it out loosely and apply to the face.

The tea solution must be kept hot; not boiling of course, but hot enough to open pores and help to slide the dead cells off the skin. Taking enough time is part of the secret. While it helps, of course, however long you do it, 15 minutes seems to give the best results.

What is the magic here? The skin truly does become new. The tea contains the papaya enzyme, which actually dissolves the dead debris on the skin that prevents the living layer beneath from renewing itself. This frees the living complexion below.

You have to experience this papaya treatment to believe the excellent results. You will marvel that your skin can feel and look the same as it did many years earlier, merely from using this treatment. The complexion actually takes on the texture and appearance of fine porcelain after the piled-up debris of dead cells has been removed. And it is entirely safe—even for people with skin disturbances. Not only does it beautify, but the warm compresses of the astringent tea seem to improve certain skin disorders.

Another preparation used in many places around the world is the standby, oatmeal, applied to the skin as a powder, as a paste, and as a dry cleaner.

In using oatmeal in its finest form, mix two tablespoons of oat flour with enough water to make a smooth paste. Wet the face and hands, then pat the oat paste over the face. (Hands, too, if you wish. It also helps them.) Leave it on the skin for several minutes, then rinse the paste off with warm, then cool water, and dry with patting motions.

To use oatmeal as a dead skin debris remover, add two tablespoons of oats to one-half cup of cold milk. Bring the mixture to an easy boil and cook until you have a soft meal. Add one tablespoon of rose water. Allow the oatmeal to cool, then spread it on the face and neck. After 15 minutes, rinse it off with warm and then cool water, and pat the skin dry with a very clean cloth or facial tissues.

To use oatmeal as a dry cleanser, simply stand over a basin and rub a dry, fine oatmeal over every part of your face, except the eye areas. *Never* rub the skin around the eyes.

The old favorite, corn meal, still works wonders, though it is really for pretty dire cases, where a facial for removing dead cells hasn't been used in a long time, if ever. This should not be used on irritated skin. Because it is dry and granular, and less given to softening by liquid than oatmeal, the corn meal should be prepared in advance and left to soak a bit in warm water. This will reduce its coarseness and avoid damaging a too-sensitive skin.

Mix one-fourth cup of corn meal with enough warm water to make a paste. This is then applied to the face and neck in uplifting motions. Allow the paste to dry on the skin, then rub it off with a clean washcloth, or

[185]

tissues. Rinse the face and neck with warm and then cool water.

After the corn meal treatment, your skin will probably be tinged with pinkness from the friction, and you'll see pores you didn't know were there.

Almond meal for cleansing the face is popularly used in Spain, and in Portugal, where the almond trees grow.

If you do have any difficulty in finding the almond meal, it is easy enough to make it right in your kitchen. Just toss a handful of raw, unblanched almonds into the blender, and within seconds you will have a quantity of the finest meal.

This powdery meal can then be made into a paste by adding a little water, applied to the face and neck, and allowed to dry. Afterwards, using a fresh washcloth, rub gently at the surface skin, creating the friction necessary to remove the dead cells.

It is all according to your own needs. If you have taken fairly good care of your skin, then perhaps you want only a gentle friction to loosen the dead cells and bring it to top shape. But if neglect has led to an accumulation of lifeless skin that makes you appear years older than you are, then by all means use these various kinds (not all at once, of course) of cleansing agents.

Anything that induces friction should not be applied to an inflamed and infected skin. However herbal teas, such as the papaya tea, act as an astringent and draw out the toxins beneath the surface.

Finally, there is the matter of sleep. When you fail

to sleep well for several days, your face tells the story: the skin is pale, the muscles taut and unattractive, the hollows beneath the cheeks more pronounced, with dark, heavy bags under the eyes. Sometimes the skin even becomes dry and seems totally lifeless.

If you have trouble getting to sleep, an excellent approach to relaxation is described by Dr. Edmund Jacobson in his book *You Can Sleep Well* (McGraw-Hill). Jacobson points out that relaxing requires release of tension not only in the arms and legs, but in the breathing apparatus, forehead and brow, eyes and speech muscles. These are his instructions:

"Lie comfortably in bed, have no part of your body bearing on another, not even an arm or hand under your head . . . You'll find that your eyes and mouth, your forehead, cheeks, and your general muscular structure are tense. Let go, putting your entire weight on the bed. Don't let any of your weight be supported by your muscles.

"Next brake your racing thoughts by thinking positively and exclusively about your breathing. Concentration on your breathing will take all of your attention and drive out all other mental activity. By practicing total relaxation of body and mind, you'll soon experience a pleasant, floating sensation, well on your way to that first stage of sleep."

Here's a quick exercise to help you tone up as well as to relax you for sleeping: Stand straight and tall. Raise your arms at the sides to shoulder height. Keeping your arms stiff, rotate them in small circles, first clockwise, then counter-clockwise. This relieves the tight feeling across arms, shoulders and neck.

If excess tension and an excessively active mind are keeping you awake nights, jogging an hour before bedtime may be good for you. The body and mind are interrelated, and the comfortable weariness that follows strenuous exercise is often the perfect sleeping pill. If a brisk walk does the trick for you, so much the better.

After following a sensible daily exercise program for only a month, you'll find yourself facing each day with a smile instead of a growl, for you've created your own magical sleeping potion. Why become enslaved by a barbiturate or a vibrating bed? It makes much better sense to let nature put you to sleep.

The next few pages supply a few additional hints about beauty care aside from nutrition, exercise and rest. Try to incorporate them into your life. The most beautiful women invariably lead full and rewarding, but simplified lives. Their approach to matters of everyday living, and their daily relationships with those around them, are not complicated by outbursts of suspicion, envy, or any other of the deadly agitations that, in time, etch themselves into the face.

They carry their practical outlook of living into their personal preparations for their best physical appearance.

We have all known women who catch the eye with a fashionable and beautifully made-up complexion. However, even with the best make-up artistry, no one's face can sustain being covered with cosmetics for a

[188]

full day without showing the results of the skin's attempts to live and breathe underneath.

Even worse for the skin is the practice of applying fresh make-up over the stale. In an emergency, a fluff of a powder puff over the nose is all you dare add. Anything more than that and you'll have a soggy pudding for a complexion.

The women who retain their smooth skin appearance the longest are usually the ones who have examined their skin carefully and know what its condition is. When the skin is oily they normalize it as much as possible. The woman who has dry skin doesn't permit her skin to remain in this state, if she cares for it. Instead, she brings her complexion around to a more normal condition by her treatment of it. The important thing is to analyze your skin. Do it with a magnifying make-up mirror. Check for resiliency of the skin, for dryness, for troublespots. Then go to work.

There are many approaches to caring for one's skin. It is fun to experiment with natural skin care, to try various recipes, and to note the change or improvements that come about. It is also safe, because when you use a natural approach to beauty, you are merely extending the good care of nutrition to the outside of your body. The face can benefit from exterior application of nourishing food much more than it can from chemical or commercially chemicalized products.

Oily skin is a frequent complaint. To keep such a skin in good condition requires more frequent cleansing because of the inclination for make-up to mix with skin oils and clog the pores. Never use hot water on your face or body for general bathing. Though durable, the skin is still a fragile covering, and heavy handed assaults on it will do nothing to improve any condition.

For cleansing oily skin, use warm water, a non-alkaline soap, and if you have one, a complexion brush. Good circulation under skin tissues means the battle for healthy skin is half won.

Gently pat lather into the oily skin with brush, washcloth or hand, covering your forehead, chin, cheeks and neck. Rinse several times in warm, then in cool water. Pat dry with a clean towel. Next use a mixture of one tablespoon of apple-cider vinegar to one-third cup of cold water and splash on the face. Pat dry.

Results can be noticed immediately from the vinegar rinse. The skin seems to pull together more firmly and becomes fresher. This is an ancient remedy for many cosmetic ills.

For dry skins, there are many treaments. A simple one, and a growing favorite in this country, is mayonnaise. Not salad dressing, for it is the ingredients that count—the eggs, oil, and lemon juice.

Each day rub in enough to cover the entire face and neck. The neck is as susceptible as the face to the wrinkles that dry skin seems to bring on.

Leave the mayonnaise on for a minimum of 15 minutes. This treatment works better if it is left on double that time. Don't miss a day. If you apply this as soon as you arise in the morning, after a while it becomes a regular routine. It can be rinsed off after breakfast. If you don't go to work, then by all means wait until you're alone. Shortly after it is applied, the mayonnaise is absorbed into the skin. Rinse with warm, then cool water.

Before applying make-up, try one of the cooking oils as a foundation. Cold-pressed olive oil is an almost perfect lotion to be used beneath a powder base. Place a thin coat of the oil over the face and neck by patting in gently. With both hands filled with warm water, rinse over and over. You'll feel the oil smoothing out on your skin as the warm water causes it to spread. Some women benefit by the apple-cider vinegar and water rinse used after the oil.

Olive oil has long been used to smooth dry complexions. While it is more beneficial to work at this problem from within, great results can come from external application of oils and creams which give a protective coating to the skin.

These home-beauty formulas have endured for generations—some for centuries!—and are still preferred by many wealthy women who can afford the latest, most expensive beauty preparations. Their endurance is anchored in the most basic appeal—they *work*. And more than that, from a health point of view, they are safe. Dozens of recipes for the secret potions that women have employed for beauty since Cleopatra's time compare favorably with products offered by sophisticated cosmetic counters in the swankiest department stores. It is easy enough for a curious woman to test some of the recipes with what she has on hand.

If nothing else would get today's woman to try mixing her own beauty aids, the prices of the commercial

[191]

cosmetics might drive her to it. Actually, the ingredients in any cream or lotion cost only a few pennies, sometimes a fraction of a cent. What the patrons pay for is expensive packaging and advertising, plus unreasonable profits.

Cosmetics can and should be "good enough to eat." Dr. Glen J. Sperandio, associate professor of pharmacy at Purdue University showed that natural foods are not only danger-free cosmetics, but also as effective as the available commercial products and, in some instances, more beneficial. The exhibits included an effective anti-chapping cream made from tapioca, and a complexion lotion concocted from fresh peaches and cream.

Basically a woman is prepared to fight the beauty wars if she is armed with some or all of the following: the juice from melons, lemons, cucumbers, strawberries and even green beans; eggs, honey, milk, cream and buttermilk; oatmeal, almond meal, bran and barley; coconut oil, olive oil, castor oil, almond oil; the fats from animals and extracts from flowers, herbs, and other plants.

Raw egg white, used externally as a beauty mask, is one of the oldest and most effective beauty treatments known. All you do is clean your face and then smear it with raw egg white. Leave it on for 10 minutes—or longer, then rinse it off with tepid water. You can feel it drawing impurities out of your skin, tightening it and closing the pores. After you remove it, your skin is baby soft, looks clean and fresh and feels wonderful.

[192]

How do you get your face really clean? Use olive oil, glycerine or even baby oil. Just smooth on, then wipe your face with a facial tissue or absorbent cotton, being sure to get *all* of the oil off.

The shower bath is the modern, quick way to keep fresh, but the luxury of a hot, leisurely tub bath is hard to beat. You may want to experience an herb-vinegar bath, said to tone your skin and refresh your spirits: take 2 drams of rosemary, rue, lavender and camphor, soak them in a pint of white wine vinegar for several hours; strain off the herbs and add the liquid to the bath water.

You don't have to be a nut to pursue beauty the natural way: Marlene Deitrich pampers her face, neck and hands with pure lanolin lotion. Joan Crawford relaxes with wet tea bags on her eyes to brighten and rest them. The late Grace Moore, Metropolitan Opera star and movie beauty, used to rub castor oil on her face and neck every day. (This is a trick of many actresses— olive oil is also a favorite—to keep wrinkles away.) Gloria Swanson uses raw fruit and vegetables (cucumbers, strawberries, peaches) on her face.

Clearly women can make the most of their looks without resorting to dangerous cosmetic products.

Index

A

Abstracta Dermatologica, 118
Acidity, 68-70, 169
Acne, 1, 11, 103-112, 145
 lotions for, 163
 salt and, 111
 vitamin A acid and, 26, 105-108
 vitamin C and, 109
 vitamin D and, 108-109
Acne rosacea, 110
Acta. Med. Scandinav, 176
ACTH, 126
Acute hepatitis, 32
Air pollution, 2, 73
 asthma, 75
 eczema, 75-76
Air-conditioning, 54-55
Alexander, Suzanne, 174
Alkalinity, 68-70, 169
"All About Acne" (Bairstow), 110
Allergies, 1-2, 59
 air pollution, 73, 75-76
 clothes, 64-67
 detergents, 70-73
 earrings, 77
 glass fiber materials, 76
 menthol, 76-77
 perfume, 57-58, 162
 pets, 77
 rubber, 74
 shoes, 60-64
 soap, 67-70
Almond meal, as facial treatment, 184-185
Alpha tocopherol, *see* Vitamins
American Association for the Advancement of Science, 23
American Dermatological Association, 59
American Dermatological Society, 2
American Institute of Hypnosis, 176
American Journal of Diseases of Children, The, 118

American Medical Association, 26, 88, 110, 156
 Book of Health, 173
 Committee on Cosmetics, 175
 Journal of, 25, 36, 64, 66, 74, 130-131, 144
American Practitioner and Digest of Treatment, 72
Amino acids, 129
Aminophenols, 160
Aminopyrine, 146
Amodiaquine, 146
Angioma, spider, 32-33
Aniline dyes, 160
Antibiotics, 164
Antihistamines, 39, 145
Antiperspirants, 56, 58
Antipyrines, 146
Archives of Dermatology and Syphilology, 62, 77, 108, 136
Archives of Research, 12
Aron, 24
Ashe, W. F., 55
Aspirin, 146-147
Asthma, 20
 air pollution and, 75
Athlete's foot, 61, 70
 causes, 113-115
 treatment, 115-116
Atopic dermatitis, 147
Aureomycin, 38
Avitaminosis, 11

B

B complex, *see* Vitamins
Bacitracin, 164
Baer, Rudolph L., 10, 11, 144, 166
Bairstow, Bruce, 110-111
Baldness, 30, 171, 172-176
Bamford, J. A. C., 95, 97
Barbiturates, 146
Barden, Robert P., 139
Bathing, 58, 67-69

Beauty plan
  cleanliness, 181-185
  diet, 178
  exercise, 179-181
  natural cosmetics, 182-185, 188-192
  sleep, 185-187
Bechet, P., 126
Becker, S. William, Jr., 42, 115
Beeson, W. M., 141
Behrman, Howard T., 173, 174
Benzoyl peroxide, 26, 107
Besnier's prurigo, 119-122
Bettey, F. Ray, 68
Bicknell, 117
Bile, 32
Biochemical Journal, 134
Birth control pills, *see* Oral contraceptives
Bithionol, 146
Blackheads, 5, 103
Blisters, 4-5, 83
  fever, 20
Blood sugar, 28-29
Blood vessels, 6-7
Bluefarb, Samuel M., 32, 109
Boils, 14, 27
Bommer, Sigwald, 13-15
Book of Health (American Medical Association), 173
Bourgeois-Spinasse, Mme., 175
Brain, Reginald T., 5-6
Brewer's yeast, 17, 110, 131, 134, 138, 152
British Journal of Dermatology, The, 48
British Medical Journal, 100
Brodie, Sheldon, 10, 11
Bromides, 145, 146
Bruising, 2, 4
Bryan, William J., Jr., 176
Burks, James W., 158, 162
Burns, 83-93
  children and, 92-93
  classification, 83
  first aid measures, 88
  FRST, 90-91
  protein and, 84
  salt and, 87
  shock due to, 84
  vitamin C and, 84
  vitamin E and, 85-87
Butter yellow, 165

C

Calcium, 101, 168
Calcium carbonate, 46, 48
Callouses, 5
Camarron, Charles S., 41
Canadian Medical Association Journal, 19-20, 68, 168
Cancer, *see* Skin cancers
Capillaries, 7
Cappon, D., 19-20
Carbohydrates, 16
Carbon tetrachloride, 165
Caro, William A., 32
Carotene, 118-119
Carruthers, Ronald, 47
Castor oil, 89
Chapping, 70
Cheilosis, 10
Chicken-pox, 97, 102
Children
  burns and, 92-93
  eczema and, 2, 13, 15, 117, 118, 121, 122
  prickly heat and, 79-80
Chlorpromazine, 146
Cirrhosis, 32-33
Clairol, Inc., 160
Cleanliness, 58, 67-69, 181-185
Clinical Medicine, 141
Clinical Toxicology of Commercial Products, 56, 160
Clothes, contact dermatitis and, 65-67
Cluver, E. H., 46, 48
Coal tar, 152, 159
Cocoa butter, 49
Cod liver oil, 89
Cold sores, 20
Colds, 96
Comedones, 105-106
Contact dermatitis, 2, 59
  air pollution, 73, 75-76
  clothes, 65-67
  detergents, 70-73
  earrings, 77
  glass fiber materials, 76
  menthol, 76-77
  pets and, 77
  rubber, 74
  shoes, 60-64
  soaps, 67-70
Corn meal, as facial treatment, 184
Cornstarch, 19, 30, 58

Cornell University, Clinical Nutritional Unit, 129
Cortisone, 126-127, 145
Cosmetics, 19, 156-167
  face creams, 161-162
  for fingernails, 161
  hair dyes, 159-161
  hair removers, 161
  hormone creams, 150-151, 163
  legislation, 164-167
  lipsticks, 157
  medicated, 162-164
  natural, 182-185, 188-192
  perfume, 57-58, 162
  skin cancer, relation to, 164-165
Costello, M. J., 136
Coursin, David, 101
Craig, Marjorie, 179-181
Crawford, Joan, 192
Cyclamates, 37-38
Cytosine arabioside, 100

D

Dandruff, 126, 171-172
Daniels, Farrington, Jr., 37
Davidson, Charles S., 16
DDT, 162
Dehydration exhaustion, 53
Deitrich, Marlene, 192
Denver Post, 76
Deodorants, 56-58
Dermis, 4, 6-8, 43
Dessicated liver, 17, 131, 134, 138
Detergents, 68, 70-73
Diabetes, 33
Diathetic Besnier's prurigo, 119-122
Diet, 7-8, 17, 178
  and hair, 168, 176
  protein, 16-17
  psoriasis and, 127-130, 134
  shingles and, 96, 101
  unsaturated fatty acids, 12-16
  vitiligo and, 137-138
Diffuse alopecia, 174
DNA, 153-154
Dodson, 82
Drake, Debbie, 181
Dry skin, treatment for, 189-190
Durable press fabrics, 64-67

E

Earrings, 77
Eczema, 20, 30, 117-123, 145, 147
  air pollution, 75-76
  children and, 2, 13, 15, 117, 118, 121, 122
  diathetic Besnier's prurigo, 119-122
  housewives', 72
  soy products, 123
  unsaturated fatty acids, 13-15, 117-118
  vitamin A, 118
  vitamin B, 119-122
  vitamin B, 117
Edema, 150
Edgerton, Milton T., 42
Edmundson, Walter F., 162
Effect of Continued Exposure to Air Pollution on Incidence of Chronic Childhood Disease (Sultz), 75
Egyptian Pharmaceutical Bulletin, 124
Emotions, 19-21
Engmen, Martin F., Jr., 72
Epidermis, 4-6, 37, 43, 75, 181
Epstein, Ernst, 57-58, 60-62, 64
Erythema, multiple, 30
Erythema, palmar, 33
Estrogen, 143-144, 150-151, 163
Exercise, 178
  facial, 179-181
  in heat, 54-56
  isometric, 179-181
  isotonic, 179
  sleep and, 186
Eye, Ear, Nose and Throat Monthly, The, 158

F

Face creams, 161-162
Face lifts, 151
Facial exercises, 179-181
Facial treatments
  almond meal, 184-185
  corn meal, 184
  oatmeal, 183-184
  papaya, 182-183
Fever blisters, 20

INDEX

Findley, G. H., 47
Fingernails, 5, 6
  hardener, 161
  polish, 161
Fish oil, 17
Flesch, P., 48
Fluorescent lighting, dermatitis and, 39-40
Fluorides, 147-149
Foldes, Eugene, 175
Folic acid, 15
Food, Drug and Cosmetic Act (1938), 159
Food additives, 11
Food and Drug Administration, 91, 133, 165, 166
Formaldehyde, 65
Formalin, 65
Francis, H. W., 135
Frank, Benjamin S., 152-155
Free radicals, 37
Freeman, Joel S., 141
Frost, Phillip, 25, 131-132
FRST, 90-91
Fulton, James E., Jr., 26, 106. 107
Fusaro, Dr. Ramon M., 39-40

G

Gaul, Edward, 111
General Practitioner, 42, 73
George, J. Otto, 89-91
Glass fiber materials, 76
Glycogen, 28-29
Gold sodium thiomalate, 146
Goodman, Herman, 172
Gottlob, Milford, 144
Grabner, H., 30
Griseofulvin, 146
Gross, Paul, 127-128
Gupta, A. K., 100

H

Hair, 5-6, 168-177
  baldness, 30, 171, 172-176
  dandruff, 126, 171-172
  diet, 168, 176
  dyes, 159-161
  follicles, 5, 28, 170
  growth rate, 171
  permanent waving, 169, 174

  pigment, 170-171
  protein, 168-169
  removers, 161
  shampoos, 169-170, 172
  straighteners, 174
Halibut liver oil, 133
Harris, Harriet, 144
Heat, exercise in, 54-56
Heat exhaustion, 52-53
Heat stroke, 53-54
Hemochromatosis, 33
Henderson, 35-36
Hepatitis, acute, 32
Herpes zoster, *see* Shingles
Hexachlorophene, 36
Hindson, T. C., 30, 79-82
Hives, 146-147
Hormone creams, 150-151, 163
Hormones, 143-145
Hudson, A. L., 68
Hydrochloric acid, 135
Hyman, Daniel, 139
Hyperkeratosis, *see* Warts
Hypnosis, baldness and, 176

I

Ichthyosis, 2, 10, 124-125
  Lamellar, 26
  vitamin A acid and, 25-26, 131-132
Impetigo, 14
Indian Practitioner, The, 100
Industrial Medicine and Surgery, 162
Interferon, 23
International Institute for Age Therapy, 151
Iodides, 145, 146
Isometric exercises, 179-181
Isotonic exercises, 179

J

Jacobson, Edmund, 185-186
Jaundice, 32
Johnson, Brian E., 37
Jolles, K. E., 100
Josephs, 24
Journal of the American Dietetic Association, 117

[198]

Journal of the American Medical Association, 25, 36, 64, 66, 74, 130-131, 144
Journal of the American Medical Women's Association, 174, 175
Journal of Chiba Medical Society, 27
Journal of the Indiana State Medical Association, The, 111
Journal of Investigative Dermatology, 130
Journal of Nutrition, 24
Journal of Pediatrics, 133
Journal of the Southern Medical Association, 158

K

Kagan, B. M., 24-25
Kalivas, James, 36
Kane, Sidney, 123
Kansas State Department of Health, 105
Kennedy, C. B., 66-67
Keratosis, 30, 44, 106
Kerlan, Irvin, 165
Kesten, Beatrice M., 117, 127-128
Kirk, 165, 166
Klenner, Fred, 98
Kligman, Albert, 44, 107
Kline, Paul, 109
Knutson, Gunilla, 181
Krehl, W. A., 2, 101, 117
Kuhn, B. H., 140

L

Lactoflavine, 121, 122
LaLanne, Jack, 181
Lamellar ichthyosis, 26
Lancet, The, 31, 36, 41, 63, 67, 79, 103
Lanolin, 162, 192
Lawrie, 24
Lazar, Paul, 156
Leather, in shoes, 62-64
Lecithin, 123, 127-128, 134
Lee Foundation Report, 118
Lehigh County (Pa.) Medical Society, 113
LeShay, Philip, 141

Lewis, J. M., 133
Linoleic acids, 13, 14
Linolenic acids, 13, 14
Lipsticks, 157
Liver, dessicated, 17, 131, 134, 138
Liver diseases, 32, 33
Liver extract, 109
London Institute of Dermatology, 42
Lowney, Edmund D., 104
Lubowe, Irwin I., 3, 73
Lung diseases, 33
Lye, 164

M

McClure, James, Jr., 101
McGowan, E. M., 76
Madden, John F., 130
Magnesium, 101
Malaria rubra papulosa, see Prickly heat
Marshal, Wallace, 109
Maynard, Merlin, 108, 130
Medical Clinics of North America, The, (Krehl), 2
Medical Journal of Australia, 95, 97
Medical Science, 123
Medical Times, 117
Medical Tribune, 144
Melanin, 43
Menopause, 150-151
Menthol, 76-77
Mercaptobenzthiazole, 61-62
Merck Manual, 96
Mercurials, 145
Minnesota Medicine, 39
Mital, H. S., 100
Molnar, Joseph A., 95-96
Moore, 24, 192
Moore-Robinson, Miriam, 147
Morris, George E., 109
Multiple erythema, 30
Munchener Medizinische Wochenschrift (Munich Medical Weekly), 13, 30
Murphy, R. J., 55

INDEX

N

Nails, 5, 6
  hardeners, 161
  polishes, 161
Nation, The, 164
"Natural History of Herpes Zoster" (Bamford), 95, 97
Neomycin, 145
Neomycin sulfate, 164
Nerves, 6
New England Journal of Medicine, 101
New Hope for Your Skin (Lubowe), 3
New Scientist, The, 68
New York State Journal of Medicine, 87
Niacin (vitamin B₃), 8, 124-125
Nucleic acids, 152-155
Nutrition, *see* Diet; Vitamins
Nutrition Today, 101

O

Oatmeal, as facial treatment, 183-184
Oily skin, treatment for, 188-189
O'Quinn, E. E., 66-67
Oral contraceptives, 36, 38, 145
  as acne treatment, 104
Orentreich, Norman, 174, 175

P

Palmar erythema, 33
Pancreatic disease, 33-34
Pantothenic acid, 128-168
Papaya treatment, 182-183
Para-amino-benzoic acid (PABA), 136-138
Paradiaminobenzenes, 160
Paraphenylenediamine, 64, 159
Patiala, R., 119-121
Patterson, Clara E., 181
Pauling, Linus, 96
Pellagra, 8, 20
Penicillin, 146, 164
Peroxides, 37
Perfume dermatitis, 57-58, 162
Perlenfein, Harold H., 169

Permanent waving, 169, 174
Pets, allergies and, 77
pH, 69
Phenolphthalein, 146
Phenylbutazone, 146
Phillips, Clarence, 89
Phosphoric acid, 168
Phosphorus, 101
Photodermatoses, 156-157
Photosensitivity, 35-40, 59, 146
Physiological Review, 48
Pigments, 32, 170-171
Pillsbury, 115
Pitts, Ferris, Jr., 101
Platou, Ralph V., 68
Politzer, 48
Polyarthritis, 33
Polymyxin, 164
Porphia, 33
Porphyria cutanea tarda, 143-144
Postgraduate Medicine, 95
Potassium, 54, 87-88
Potassium dichromate, 62-63
Practitioner, The (Baer, Brodie) 10
Prescott, 117
Press Medicale, 175
Prevention Magazine, 48, 113, 147
Prickly heat, vitamin C and, 30, 79-82
Progesterone, 150
Protein, 7-8, 11, 16-17, 54
  burns and, 84
  hair and, 168-169
  taurine in, 129-130
Psoriasis, 14, 15, 20, 125-134
  diet, 127-130, 134
  lecithin and, 127-128, 134
  taurine and, 129, 130
  vitamin A acid and, 25-26, 131-133
  vitamin B and, 130-131
Pyridoxine (vitamin B₆), 2, 29, 117, 128

R

Rashes, 59-78
  See also Allergies
Resorcin, 163
Riboflavin (vitamin B₂), 2, 8, 10, 29, 128, 168
  eczema and, 119-122
  psoriasis and, 130

Richards, Ralph C., 67
RNA, 153-154
Rodale, J. I., 113, 114
Roe, Daphne A., 7, 8, 128-130
Roenigk, Henry H., 144
Rothman, Stephen, 163, 164
Rubber sensitivity, 61-62, 64

S

St. John's Hospital for Diseases of
    the Skin, 42
Salicylates, 146
Salt
    acne and, 111
    baldness and, 175-176
    burns and, 87
Sandler, Marvin, 140
Scabies, 77
Schizophrenia, 20
Schneider, 12
Scientific American, 37
Scotchguard, 67
Scurvy, 11
Sebaceous glands, 5, 6, 75, 105, 106,
    171-172
Seborrhea, 171-172
Sebum, 5, 105, 106
Shampoos, 168-170, 172
Sharman, 24
Shelley, Walter B., 74
Shingles, 96-102
    diet and, 96, 101
    vitamin B_{12} and, 96, 100
    vitamin C and, 96, 98-99
Shock, due to burns, 84
Shoes, contact dermatitis and, 60-64
Shute, Wilfred E., 85-86
Sidi, Edwin, 175
Sieve, Benjamin, 135-138
Skin cancers, 2, 18, 41, 42
    cosmetics and, 164-165
Skin Diseases (Brain), 6
Skin syphilis, 30
Skin tuberculosis, 30
Sleep, 178, 185-187
Soap, 18, 19, 67-70, 105
    anti-bacterial, 36, 38
    photosensitivity and, 36, 38
Society of Cosmetic Chemists, 163
Society of Toxicology, 156
Sodium, 87-88
Sodium chloride, 54

South African Medical Journal, 46,
    48
Southern Medical Journal, 140
Southern Medicine and Surgery, 98
Soy milk, 123
Soybean lecithin, 127
Soybeans, 123, 130
Sperandio, Glen J., 190
Spider angioma, 32-33
Staphylococcus organisms, 27
Steroid drugs, 25, 99, 126-127
Stokes, 115
Straumfjord, Jon D., 108
Strauss, Sara Mildred, 181
Subdermis, 4
Sulfides, 161
Sulfonamides, 38, 146
Sulfonylureas, 146
Sulfur resorcinal, 107
Sullivan, Leonor K., 165-166
Sultz, Harry A., 75
Sunflower seeds, 17
Suntan, 18, 19, 41-51
    anti-sunburn pill, 46-48
    lotions, 45-46, 49
    photosensitivity and, 35-37, 39
Swanson, Gloria, 192
Sweat glands, 3, 5, 6, 82
Sweating, 52-58

T

Takenouchi, Katsu, 27-30
Tappel, A. L., 37
Taub, S. J., 158, 162
Taurine, 129-130
Temperature, 3
Terramycin, 38
Tetrachlorosalicylanilide, 146
Tetracycline, 104
Tetramethylthiuram sulphide, 62
Thiamine (vitamin B_1), 29, 30, 128,
    130-131
Thiazide diuretics, 38
Thioglycolic acid, 161
Thiram, 74
Thomas, Virginia Castleton, 48
Thompson, Betty, 35
Thompson, John, 35
Time Magazine, 72
Today's Health, 110
Toenails, 5
Toilet Goods Association, 166

INDEX

Toxic epidermal necrolysis, 145
Tranquilizers, photosensitivity and, 36
Trypsin, 123
Tulipan, Louis, 110
Tyrothricin, 164

U

Ulcers (external), 14, 15
University of Utah Review, 67
Unsaturated fatty acids, 11-16
  eczema and, 117-118
Urea formaldehyde resins, 65-66
Uroporphyrin, 143
Urticaria, 147

V

Van der Leun, Jan C., 37
Van der Nerwe, L. W., 48
Van Scott, Eugene J., 164, 167
Varicella-zoster virus, 97
Viruses, 23, 30
"Vitamin E for Ailing and Healthy
  Hearts" (Shute), 85
Vitamins
  A, 2, 17, 134, 142, 168
    in anti-sunburn pill, 46-48
    eczema and, 118
    infection and, 22-25
    warts and, 140-141
    wound healing, 25
  A acetate, 131
  A acid
    acne and, 11, 26, 105-108
    ichthyosis, 25-26, 131-132
    psoriasis and, 25-26, 131-133
  A alcohol, 131
  A aldehyde, 131
  A palmitate, 140-141
  B₁ (thiamin), 29, 30, 128
    psoriasis and, 130-131
  B₂ (riboflavin), 2, 8, 10, 29, 128, 168
    eczema and, 119-122
    psoriasis and, 130
  B₃ (niacin), 8, 124-125
  B₆ (pyridoxine), 2, 29, 117, 128
  B₁₂, 30, 168
    psoriasis and, 131
    shingles and, 96, 100

C, 2, 17
  acne and, 109
  burns and, 84
  colds and, 96
  prickly heat and, 30, 79-82
  shingles and, 96, 98-99
  vitiligo and, 136
D, 127, 133, 134
  acne and, 108-109
E (alpha tocopherol), 14-15, 133
  burns and, 85-87
Vitamins in Medicine (Bicknell, Prescott), 117
Vitiligo, 135-138
Von Beer, 132

W

Warin, Robert P., 147
Warts, 139-142
Water, fluoridation of, 147-149
Weinstein, Gerald D., 25, 131-132
Wet Bulb Temperature Guide, 55-56
Wheat germ, 14, 15, 134, 138
Whiteheads, 5
Wilhelmi, Charles M., 95
Witten, Victor, 173
Wolf, George, 22
Worne, 12
Wrinkles, 16-17, 150-155, 179

X

X-ray
  as acne treatment, 104
  as psoriasis treatment, 126

Y

Yeast, 152
You Can Sleep Well (Jacobson), 185-186
Your Hair (Goodman), 172

Z

Zawahry, M. R., 124-125